Faith in Freedom

Books by Thomas Szasz

Pain and Pleasure
The Myth of Mental Illness
Law, Liberty, and Psychiatry
Psychiatric Justice
The Ethics of Psychoanalysis
The Manufacture of Madness
Ideology and Insanity
The Age of Madness (ed.)
The Second Sin
Ceremonial Chemistry
Heresies
Karl Kraus and the Soul Doctors
Schizophrenia
Psychiatric Slavery
The Theology of Medicine
The Myth of Psychotherapy
Sex by Prescription
The Therapeutic State
Insanity
The Untamed Tongue
Our Right to Drugs
A Lexicon of Lunacy
Cruel Compassion
The Meaning of Mind
Fatal Freedom
Pharmacracy
Liberation by Oppression
Words to the Wise
Faith in Freedom

Faith in Freedom

Libertarian Principles and Psychiatric Practices

Thomas Szasz

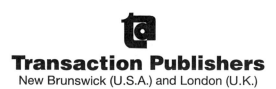

Transaction Publishers
New Brunswick (U.S.A.) and London (U.K.)

First paperback printing 2015
Copyright © 2004 by Transaction Publishers, New Brunswick, New Jersey.

This book is printed on acid-free paper that meets the American National Standard for Permanence of Paper for Printed Library Materials.

Library of Congress Catalog Number: 2003066308
ISBN: 978-0-7658-0244-6 (cloth); 978-1-4128-5577-8 (paper)
Printed in the United States of America

Library of Congress Cataloging-in-Publication Data

Szasz, Thomas Stephen, 1920-
    Faith in freedom : libertarian priciples and psychiatric practices / Thomas Szasz.
                p.   cm.
    Includes bibliographical references and index.
    ISBN 978-1-4128-5577-8
    1. Psychiatric ethics. 2. Medical ethics. 3. Patients—Legal status, laws, etc. I. Title.
[DNLM: 1. Psychiatric—ethics. 2. Patient Rights. 3. Personal Autonomy. WM 100 S996f 2004]
RC455.2.E8S98 2004
174'.2—dc22   2003066308

Our faith in freedom does not rest on the foreseeable results in particular circumstances, but on the belief that it will, on balance, release more forces for the good than for the bad.... Freedom granted only when it is known beforehand that its effects will be beneficial is not freedom.

Friedrich von Hayek (1899-1992)
The Constitution of Liberty[1]

Contents

C. Libertarians

Preface

There often comes a time in human affairs when some people believe, deeply and sincerely, that certain ideas and practices—with far-reaching economic, moral, and political consequences—are right, while others believe, just as deeply and sincerely, that these ideas and practices are wrong. For a long time, chattel slavery was such an idea. Today, it is psychiatric slavery.

"I am the Lord thy God, which have brought thee out of the land of Egypt, out of the house of bondage" (Exodus, 20: 2; King James version). So reads the First Commandment. Note that God does not say: "I am the Lord thy God, which have abolished the institution of bondage for all mankind." On the contrary, the Old Testament recognizes slavery as a social institution and, by not condemning it, legitimizes it: "Both thy bondmen, and thy bondmaids, which thou shalt have, shall be of the heathen that are round about you; of them shall ye buy bondmen and bondmaids" (Leviticus, 25: 44; King James version).

For millennia, slavery was a universally accepted human relationship: it was the slave's duty to serve his master, and the master's duty to care for his slave. The abolitionists had to face and overcome this image of slavery as protection for the slave, bolstered by benevolence, care, and security as the moral building blocks of a revered institution. They did not argue that abolition would satisfy the needs of slaves better than did slavery. Instead, they maintained that individual liberty is a transcendent moral value that renders involuntary servitude—regardless of any good in it, real or attributed—immoral and illegitimate. The abolitionist response to the outrage of involuntary servitude was the abolition of slavery, not its reform.

Today, psychiatric slavery—that is, the coercive control of the patient by the psychiatrist—is all but universally regarded as an integral part of sound medical practice and civilized social life. For nearly fifty years I have argued that this view is medically unfounded and morally unacceptable.[1] Instead of restating my case against the subjection of mental patients to psychiatrists, I cite John Stuart Mill's reflections about the obstacles he faced in presenting his case against the tradition-sanctioned subjection of women to men. In 1869, in *The Subjection of Women,* he wrote:

> So long as an opinion is strongly rooted in the feelings...the worse it fares in argumentative contest, the more persuaded its adherents are that their feeling must have some deeper ground, which the arguments do not reach; and while the feeling remains, it is always throwing up fresh intrenchments of argument to repair any breach in the old.... [T]he understandings of the majority of mankind would need to be much better cultivated than has ever yet been the case, before they can be asked to place such reliance in their own power of estimating arguments, as to give up practical principles in which they have been born and bred and which are the basis of much of the existing order of the world, at the first argumentative attack which they are not capable of logically resisting.[2]

The Declaration of Independence states: "We hold these truths to be self-evident, that all men are created equal, that they are endowed by their Creator with certain unalienable Rights, that among these are Life, Liberty and the pursuit of Happiness." Prior to the Civil War, classifying black men and women as property, not persons ("men"), rendered slavery compatible with a free society. Today, classifying incarceration in a mental hospital as treatment, not punishment, renders psychiatric slavery compatible with a free society.[3]

Psychiatry has never lacked critics. Indeed, the history of psychiatry is synonymous with the history of so-called psychiatric reforms. Critics argued, and continue to argue, that their system of care for mental patients is superior to the one offered by mainstream psychiatry.

This has never been the basis of my opposition to psychiatry as a system of social control. I have steadfastly maintained that psychiatry, as we know it, must be abolished. Why? For the same reason that abolitionists maintained that slavery had to be abolished. They believed that individual liberty is a transcendent moral value that renders involuntary servitude—regardless of any good in it, real or attributed—immoral and illegitimate. I believe that involuntary psychiatry is—regardless of any good in it, real or attributed—immoral and illegitimate. The proper response to the outrage of psychiatric slavery is abolition, not reform.

I contend that this position is not merely consistent with the basic philosophy of libertarianism but is inherent in it. Unfortunately, liberty is something for which everyone regards himself as fit, but most people regard certain other persons or the members of certain groups as unfit. In the past, among the unfit were blacks, women, Jews, and "perverts" such as homosexuals. Today, the persons most often considered unfit for liberty are the mentally ill.

*   *   *

For the better part of 200 years—from 1700 to 1900—psychiatry was synonymous with the madhouse or insane asylum. All psychiatry was, *ipso facto*, involuntary psychiatry. The advent of psychoanalysis and psychotherapy toward the end of the nineteenth century brought into being two radically different kinds of mental health care existing side by side: one was asylum-based—involuntary psychiatry—a service paid for by the state (taxpayer); the other was office-based—voluntary psychiatry—a service paid for by the buyer (patient).[4] Dramatic changes in recent decades in the financing and regulation of psychiatric services led to the erosion and virtual disappearance of this important distinction.[5]

Economically, the transformation of *private psychiatry* into *public psychiatry* was brought about by shifting the cost of mental health care from the subject seeking and receiving the service to a third party (insurance company, Medicare, Medicaid) "responsible" for "covering" it. This is called "the right to psychiatric treatment." Legally, it was brought about by shifting the locus of responsibility for "harm" from the subject as moral agent to the psychiatrist as the patient's *de facto* guardian, responsible for protecting him from himself and protecting others from him. This is called "the duty to protect."

Until the 1970s, only the mental hospital psychiatrist had the duty to protect the patient from the "dangers" he posed to himself and others. (This duty was rarely enforced in practice.) The private, office-based psychiatrist—whose patient had an independent life and often occupied a social position higher than the doctor—had no such duty. The principles and practices of deinstitutionalization, outpatient commitment, the mental patient's right to treatment, and the psychiatrist's duty to protect have effectively erased the line between confined and unconfined patients; transformed all mental patients into persons actually or potentially not responsible for their actions, hence subject to psychiatric coercion; and rendered all mental health professionals responsible for their patients' misbehavior and welfare, with the duty to coerce them if necessary in their own best interest.

Famed English jurist Sir Henry Sumner Maine (1822-1888) aptly observed: "The movement of the progressive societies has hitherto been a movement *from Status to Contract.*"[6] In other words, in liberal (free) societies, the law treats persons as contracting individuals, not as members of status groups (men/women, sane/insane). Modern psychiatry has declared war on this principle. Marcia Goin, M.D., president of the

American Psychiatric Association, declares: "We can make contracts with builders, insurers, and car dealers, but not with patients."[7] Builders, insurers, and car dealers make contracts with persons whom psychiatrists call "patients." Why can't psychiatrists make contracts with them? Because contracting implies two (or more) legally equal parties, each putting his cards on the table. It implies mutual obligations, each party having legal power to compel his partner to fulfill the contract or compensate him for failure to do so.

Such mutuality is contrary to psychiatric ethics. Specifically, psychiatrists reject the "base" ethics of commerce in favor of the "loftier" ethics of care. The seller of plumbing services is obligated to deliver only that which his customer has requested and he has agreed to provide. The seller of psychiatric services is obligated to deliver much more: he must protect the customer from himself, even at the cost of depriving him of liberty.

Civilized morality and the free market presuppose a commitment to valuing cooperation and contract more highly than coercion and control. Official psychiatry declares that the ethically and legally proper practice of the profession requires the rejection of free contract in favor "therapeutic" coercion. Daniel Luchins, M.D., a professor of psychiatry at the University of Chicago, states: "[E]mphasis on protecting negative liberties may be appropriate for a society of 18th-century country squires, but not for the seriously mentally ill in the United States."[8] In other words, the psychiatrist who contracts with his patient—and fails to protect him from suicide and others from assault or murder by the patient—deviates from the "standard of psychiatric care" (is derelict in his "duty to protect" and denies the patient his "right to treatment"), and is presumed guilty of medical malpractice.[9] This is what compels all psychiatrists to function as actually or potentially coercive psychiatrists and makes noncoercive psychiatry an oxymoron.[10]

Let us not forget that there is no objective test for mental illness, much less a test to measure the severity of this alleged illness. How, then, do psychiatrists know that a mental illness is "serious"? They know it *ex post facto*: if the patient injures or kills himself or someone else, then he is said to have had a "serious mental illness." The American Constitution prohibits *ex post facto* laws. The American Psychiatric Association and American mental health laws espouse and rely on *ex post facto* determinations.

The distinguishing feature of the libertarian philosophy of freedom is the belief that self-ownership is a basic right and initiating violence is a fundamental wrong. In contrast, psychiatric practice is based on the belief that self-ownership—epitomized by suicide—is a medical wrong, and that initiating violence against persons called "mental patients" is a medical right.

Are self-medication and self-determined death exercises of rightful self-ownership, or manifestations of serious mental diseases? Does deprivation of liberty under psychiatric auspices constitute odious preventive detention, or is it therapeutically justified hospitalization? Should forced psychiatric drugging be interpreted as assault and battery or medical treatment?

How do friends of freedom—especially libertarians—deal with the conflict between elementary libertarian principles and prevailing psychiatric practices? This is the question I address and answer in the pages that follow. This book is not primarily about libertarianism or psychiatry, per se. On the contrary, it assumes that the reader possesses a measure of familiarity with both. This book is about the conflict—and incompatibility—between libertarianism and psychiatry.

Libertarians claim to be interested in issues of public policy, especially policies that infringe on individual liberty. However, they show far more interest in economic than in psychiatric policies. Libertarian conferences and publications regularly address issues such as monetary policy, taxation, regulation and deregulation, foreign aid, and welfare, but rarely, if ever, consider issues such as "civil commitment" (involuntary mental hospitalization), "outpatient commitment" (forced drugging), "psychiatric diagnosis" (accusation of dangerousness to self and others), "the insanity defense" (exculpation for a serious criminal offense, typically murder), and similar "defenses" based on "psychiatric expert testimony." While all of these policies affect the everyday lives of people, the consequences of psychiatric policies are more direct and damaging: economic policies, like civil laws, deprive people of money or economic freedom, whereas psychiatric policies, like criminal laws, deprive people of liberty or personal freedom. This is why I believe that all Americans—especially libertarians—have a moral and intellectual duty to confront the conflict between liberty and psychiatry and articulate their position regarding the idea of mental illness and the psychiatric coercions and excuses it justifies.

Admittedly, ours is an age of specialization. We expect specialists to be particularly knowledgeable about their areas of expertise and, for other matters, rely on the work of accredited experts. However, from social scientists—that is, from students of human affairs, especially if their interests encompass issues of individual liberty and personal responsibility—I believe we ought to expect more: they ought also to familiarize themselves with the few truths and many falsehoods about the medical specialty called "psychiatry." Why psychiatry? Because psychiatric interventions—in particular, civil commitment and diversions from the criminal justice to the mental health system—are the most common and most widely and uncritically accepted methods used by the modern state to deprive individuals of liberty and responsibility.

I regard psychiatry as a major threat to freedom and dignity. This is why I criticize certain libertarians not only for uncritically accepting mental health clichés that justify the psychiatric status quo, but also for averting their eyes from the conflict between liberty and psychiatry.

Neutrality in the face of evil—especially in the aftermath of the concentration camps and the Gulag—has received ample attention from historians, ethicists, and other social commentators.[11] Dante Alighieri's (1265-1321) views on the subject are worth recalling here. In the *Inferno*, Canto III, Dante introduces the reader to "The Vestibule of Hell," the place where the souls of "the Opportunists" reside. He writes: "I, holding my head in horror, cried: 'Sweet Spirit, what souls are these who run through this black haze?' And he [Virgil] to me: 'These are the nearly soulless whose lives concluded neither blame nor praise. They are mixed here with that despicable corps of angels who were neither for God nor Satan, but only for themselves. The High Creator who scourged them from Heaven and Hell will not receive them since the wicked might feel glory over them.... Mercy and Justice deny them even a name.'"[12]

*   *   *

To prevent misunderstanding or giving offense where none is intended, let it be noted that I use the plural nouns "economists" and "psychiatrists," without qualifying each time with "some" or "many," to refer to mainstream practitioners of these disciplines. I recognize that economists and psychiatrists do not all hold the same views or engage in the same practices. Similarly, when I write "economists" in reference to mathematical economists as opposed to Austrian economists, I trust that the context makes my meaning clear.[13]

There remains for me to say something about my use of the term "science." Science, from the Latin *scientia*, means knowledge. *Webster's* defines it as "possession of knowledge as distinguished from ignorance or misunderstanding; a branch or department of systematized knowledge that is or can be made a specific object of study."

The term "scientist" is a modern coinage. Persons we regard as great nineteenth-century scientists—for example, Michael Faraday (1791-1867) and Charles Darwin (1809-1882)—were not considered scientists. They were called, and called themselves, naturalists, natural philosophers, or men of science. In 1833, upon the request of poet Samuel Taylor Coleridge (1772-1834), William Whewell (1794-1866)—a Cambridge polymath widely regarded as the father of modern philosophy of science—invented the English word "scientist."[14]

We customarily distinguish between the natural sciences, exemplified by astronomy, physics, and chemistry, and the social sciences, exemplified by economics, psychology, and sociology. Many modern scientists and students of science accord the status of science only to the physical sciences, and regard the social sciences as fields of scholarly study, rather than *bona fide* sciences. Michael Polanyi wisely cautioned: "The recognition of certain basic impossibilities has laid the foundations of some major principles of physics and chemistry; similarly, recognition of the impossibility of understanding living things in terms of physics and chemistry, far from setting limits to our understanding of life, will guide it in the right direction."[15] I agree with this view.

Unavoidably, the term "science" now carries with it a heavy rhetorical baggage: calling an activity a science or scientific legitimizes it as good, rational, true, and valid, whereas withholding the term or calling the activity "unscientific" implies the opposite qualities. This may or may not be an unwarranted inference. I do not use the terms "science" and "not a science" as terms of approbation and disapprobation.

Finally, a cautionary remark about the problem of the customary use of psychiatric terms. To communicate effectively, we must use ordinary words. At the same time, we must keep in mind that ordinary words are likely to be saturated with the errors, deceptions, and self-deceptions intrinsic to customary social practices. A single illustration must suffice.

We don't call getting a speeding ticket "receiving police services"; getting audited by the Internal Revenue Service "receiving tax services"; or being indicted for a crime "receiving legal services." But we call being involuntarily diagnosed as mentally ill and incarcerated in a mental hospital "receiving mental health services."

Adherence to libertarian principles requires opposition to psychiatric slavery.

Introduction: Liberty from Psychiatry

Psychiatry is usually thought of as a healing art, a type of health care service. Sometimes it is that. However, mostly and most importantly, psychiatry is a type of social control, a legal-medical system of coercion unconstrained by the rule of law.

British psychiatrist John Crammer states: "The need to restrain the *antisocial person* leads governments to intervene both administratively and legally with these [mental] *disorders*."[1] This is not true. Governments do not "intervene with disorders," they imprison persons whom psychiatrists identify as proper subjects for such disposition. Crammer's rhetoric is characteristic of the modern psychiatrist as loyal agent of the state. First, he denies the ubiquity of psychiatric coercion: "It has not been true for 50 years that patients in mental hospitals are mostly shut up against their will." Then, he acknowledges it, distances contemporary psychiatry from it by characterizing the practice as passé, and tries to exonerate the psychiatrists from responsibility for depriving innocent persons of liberty saying that they, the psychiatrists, were "only following orders": "Nor till recently did doctors have much to say about what went on in them [mental hospitals]; they were the servants of magistrates or county councillors."[2] Today, they are creatures and servants of the state, through and through.

There is no politics without political action, no surgery without surgical action, and no psychiatry without psychiatric action. The paradigmatic psychiatric actions are civil commitment and the insanity defense, each a euphemism for depriving persons of liberty. Civil commitment—the paradigm of preventive detention—deprives the innocent individual of liberty *directly*, on the ground that he is "mentally ill and dangerous to himself or others." The insanity defense—the paradigm of the diversion of the defendant from the criminal justice system to the mental health system—deprives the person accused of lawbreaking of liberty *indirectly*, on the ground that he lacks "criminal responsibility." Imputing to the defendant mental unfitness to stand trial is a variation of this tactic. Both interventions deprive the subject of the opportunity to assert his right to trial, prove his innocence, or receive a finite prison sentence instead of an indefinite sentence in a mental hospital.[3]

Regarding the injustice intrinsic to preventive detention, British historian Lord Macaulay (Thomas Babington, 1800-1859) observed: "To punish a man because we infer from the nature of some doctrine which he holds, or from the conduct of other persons who hold the same doctrines with him, that he will commit a crime, is persecution, and is, in every case, foolish and wicked."[4]

In this connection, it is important that we not lose sight of the differences between moral responsibility and legal responsibility. Moral responsibility is independent of judicial or social sanction or the lack thereof. Innocent persons are often punished, by incarceration in prison or a mental hospital, and persons guilty of lawbreaking often go unpunished, for example, because they are not caught or charged with a crime. None of this affects their moral responsibility. Laws are made and enforced by human beings. Moral responsibility refers to accountability to a "higher law."

According to the authoritative text, *Mental Health and Law: Research, Policy, and Services* (1996), "Each year in the United States well over one million persons are civilly committed to hospitals for psychiatric treatment."[5] *The Authoritative ACLU Guide to the Rights of People with Mental Illness and Mental Retardation* doubles the number: "So in this age of deinstitutionalization, a great many people still find themselves institutionalized...admissions to all inpatient facilities for psychiatric treatment now [total] more than two million people annually."[6] The lower figure translates to more than 2,500 commitments per day. In addition, countless innocent persons are harassed by threats of commitment and involuntary treatment. The tentacles of the contemporary psychiatric slave system reach into every nook and cranny of our society, from the nursery to the nursing home.[7]

As there is no psychiatry without action deemed "psychiatric" by law and society, so there is no mental illness without action deemed "mentally ill" by law and psychiatry. Actions regarded as mentally ill are either non-criminal, like depression, in which case the libertarian code forbids initiating the use of force against (*ostensibly for*) the person; or they are criminal actions, like murder, in which case the libertarian code requires that the person be punished by penal, not psychiatric, sanctions. Regardless of whether we accept or reject mental illnesses as real diseases, non-coercive psychiatry, like non-coercive slavery, is a contradiction in terms.

Liberty: Literal and Metaphorical

The literal meaning of liberty is dyadic: freedom from external coercion. In this sense, liberty is an *interpersonal concept*, entailing two or more persons. It is freedom from control by parent, policeman, or psychiatrist. *Webster's Third New International Dictionary* defines liberty as "freedom from external restraint or compulsion," and the *Oxford English Dictionary (OED)* as "exemption or release from captivity, bondage, or slavery."

The metaphorical meaning of liberty is monadic: freedom from internal desire or passion. In this sense, liberty is an *intrapersonal concept*, entailing only one person. It is freedom from our own impulses. It is freedom from covetousness, envy, lust, insanity, mental illness. It is, in short, freedom from "self-enslavement"; it is liberty as self-control.

Philosophers and theologians have long distinguished between outer freedom and inner freedom, that is, freedom from an oppressor and freedom from our own passions or sins. Psychiatrists have appropriated this spiritual concept of freedom and founded a pseudomedical, "therapeutic" empire on it. The idea of insanity or mental illness entails the concept of unfreedom: the madman is "possessed" by "irresistible impulses" (formerly the devil), is a "victim" of "mental illness," has lost his "criminal responsibility." Hence, he is properly a ward of his kinfolk or the psychiatrist or the state.

In everyday language, we conflate and confuse these two radically different meanings of liberty, for example, when we say that for the adolescent, liberty is freedom from parents and teachers; for the prisoner, freedom from guards; for the unhappy husband or wife, freedom from marriage; for the overburdened mother, freedom from children; for the sick person, freedom from illness; for the old person, freedom from having to live. In this book, when I speak of freedom or liberty, I refer only to literal liberty, or freedom from external coercion. Freedom from our own passions is a moral, not a political, problem.

Powerful ideas—such as liberty as freely willed action, and insanity as a type of "illness" that diminishes or annuls freedom—must have deep roots in the human psyche. Those roots take their nourishment from the innate sense of free will and responsibility. From an early age, children learn to control the musculature of their bodies. With that experience comes the sense of self-control, the sense of the self as actor and agent of his own actions.

Regretting an action, we often say, "I was not myself." It's a figure of speech, a kind of apology and disavowal of the act. The phrase, "I was only following orders," made infamous by Nazi murderers, expresses a disavowal that the actor was a genuine agent of his actions, responsible for them. Both phrases articulate a claim of bondage or unfreedom, a liberty lost to the power of momentary impulses or bureaucratic superiors.

The opposite sentiment is exemplified by the legendary phrase attributed to Luther, "Here I stand. I cannot do otherwise." This striking piece of self-dramatization represents inner freedom—the affirmation of personal agency and moral responsibility—through the metaphor of feeling irresistibly compelled to follow the orders of one's own conscience (which Luther equated with God's will).

Either we follow our own inner voice or we follow the voices of others. Independence implies self-government, dependency implies enslavement to others. Lord Acton (1834-1902) put it this way: "The center and supreme object of liberty is the reign of conscience.... Liberty is the condition which makes it easy for conscience to govern."[8]

We all harbor contradictory desires and obligations, have inner conflicts, and, in a metaphorical sense, are unfree. From a political point of view, these are irrelevant considerations. Gilbert K. Chesterton (1874-1936) was right: "The madman is not the man who has lost his reason. The madman is the man who has lost everything except his reason."[9] Persons called "mental patients" are free, responsible moral agents, unless they are restrained by psychiatric representatives of the state. Like sane persons, madmen and mad women have reasons for their actions. They can and do control their behavior. If they could not do so, they would not engage in the criminal conduct in which they sometimes engage. Nor could they then be so easily controlled in insane asylums.

Everyone, at all times, is *constrained*, if not by the commands of coercers without or conscience within, then by the siren songs of tempters—luring us with political or financial power, sexual and other bodily pleasures, or creature comforts of every conceivable kind. The need to resist at least some temptations constitutes a type of constraint. Thus, *there can be no freedom from all constraints.* This may be one of the reasons why many philosophers, psychologists, psychiatrists, and neuroscientists assert that freedom of the will is an illusion.

Prevailing psychiatric doctrine and political fashion require that we regard everyone called a "mental patient" as more or less unfree. Ironically, such a person is perceived as unfree *not because he is imprisoned or otherwise controlled by psychiatrists, but because he is believed to be a "prisoner of his illness," "set free by his treatment."* According to such conventional wisdom, the person with a "diagnosable mental illness" has diminished or no control over his impulses to harm himself and others, is therefore dangerous to himself and others, and ought to be deprived of liberty and relieved of responsibility, in his own interest as well as in the interest of the community. In proportion as a person entertains this view of the mental patient, he will misperceive psychiatric agents of the state as the patient's allies, not his adversaries.

In fact, most individuals diagnosed as mentally ill do not initiate violence, while most psychiatrists routinely do just that, typically at the behest of parents, spouses, social workers, lawyers, and judges. This violence is conceptualized and accepted as "diagnosis" and "treatment."

Freedom to Do What?

The ideas of unfreedom and liberation go together in much the same way that the ideas of illness and treatment, ignorance and learning go together. We expect the doctor to heal without considering whether the patient will use his health for good or ill. We expect the teacher to educate and not concern himself with whether the student will use his learning for good or ill. We do so because we regard health and knowledge as *a priori* or absolute goods, each a *bonum in se*. This notion is the mirror image of the juridical-philosophical notion of a *malum in se*, an innately immoral act, regardless of whether it is forbidden by law, exemplified by murder. This does not mean that physicians and educators cannot question how people use health and knowledge. As moral agents, they can and indeed must do so, answer the question as they deem right, and conduct themselves accordingly.

The libertarian's situation is similar. Liberty is a *bonum in se*, a good that many people rank above health and knowledge. Liberation from coercion sets us free. To do what? The answers to this question frame the grand religious, philosophical, and political "visions" of the Good Life or the Right Way.

Set free, what shall we do? Seek the security and unfreedom of the infant or the adventure and risk-taking of the self-reliant adult? The detachment and isolation of a religious recluse or Robinson Crusoe, or the challenges of earning a living and family life?

We should reflect with the utmost care about the relationship between liberty and what we call mental illness. No one is entirely free of the prejudices of his time. Edmund Burke (1729-1797), following tradition and the law, equated madness with uncontrolled passions and "irresistible impulses" to commit mischief and took for granted that confining the madman was a good thing, for him as well as society. He famously warned: "The effect of liberty to individuals is, that they may do what they please: We ought to see what it will please them to do, before we risque congratulations, which may be soon turned into complaints.... Is it because liberty in the abstract may be classed amongst the blessings of mankind, that I am seriously to felicitate a madman, who has escaped from the protecting restraint and wholesome darkness of his cell, on his restoration to the enjoyment of light and liberty?"[10]

For a long time, while mankind was in its infancy, people regarded freedom as living in harmony with the will of the gods or God. For the devout Jew, Christian, and Muslim, liberty outside the bounds of his religion is heresy and sin. The word "islam" means "submission" (to God's will).

Politicians never tire of telling people that liberty is the natural condition of mankind, and most people have come to believe it. Modern wars are conducted under the flag of "liberation." It is a grand lie. "For thousands of years," wrote Acton, "man's history is the growth not of freedom but enslavement.... The idea that freedom is right does not loom for thousands of years."[11] That is a profound insight into the human condition, reflexively denied in the oratory of modern democratic politics. The natural condition of man appears to be submission to authority. Autonomy and liberty are psychological and political anomalies. The spirit of statism is alive and well. The rhetoric of Mussolini's celebration of "fascist" statism is the rhetoric of totalitarian democracy: "[I]f liberty is to be the attribute of the real man, and not of that abstract puppet envisaged by individualistic Liberalism, Fascism is for liberty."[12] Totalitarian democracy and the therapeutic state are also "for liberty."[13]

This salvationist-statist perspective recaptures, in an ostensibly secular imagery, the totalitarian worldview of the great monotheistic religions. In that scheme—as in Mussolini's, Hitler's, Stalin's, and psychiatry's—there is no private sphere. Everything is created by God and belongs to God. God is everywhere, regulates everything. That is why the observant Jew wears a yarmulke, a skullcap, everywhere, at all times; why the pious Catholic submits to papal infallibility; why for the devout Muslim there can be no such thing as a secular state; and why for the true believer in psychiatry there is no such thing as a psychiatry separate from the state.

British conservative social commentator, Roger Scruton, correctly observes that the Koran makes "no distinction between the public and the private spheres.... Laws governing marriage, property, usury, and commerce occur side-by-side with rules of domestic ritual, good manners, and personal hygiene. The conduct of war and the treatment of criminals are dealt with in the same tone of voice as diet and defecation.... Islam, in other words, is less a theological doctrine than a system of *piety*. To submit to it is to discover the rules for an untroubled life and an easy conscience."[14]

In a similar vein, psychiatrist G. Brock Chisholm—the highest-ranking medical officer in the Canadian Armed Forces during World War II and the first director of the World Health Organization (WHO)—declared:

> The reinterpretation and eventual eradication of the concepts of right and wrong...are the belated objectives of practically all effective psychotherapy.... If the race is to be freed of its crippling burden of good and evil it must be psychiatrists who take the original responsibility.... The world is sick and the ills are due to the perversion of man; his inability to live with himself. The microbe is not the enemy; science is sufficiently advanced to cope with it were it not for the barriers of superstition, ignorance, religious intolerance, misery, poverty.... These psychological evils must be understood that a remedy might be prescribed and the scope of the task before the Committee [Technical Preparatory Committee of the WHO] therefore knows no bounds.[15]

The prophets of the therapeutic state promise and peddle the oldest panacea devised by man—the total control of human life for the benefit of human life. Instead of entrusting unlimited power to God-and-cleric, they entrust unlimited power to therapy-and-clinician.[16] Everyone is, more or less, mentally ill and every aspect of everyone's life is the business of pharmacratic agents of the state: conservatives want to use the therapeutic state to prohibit people from doing what's bad for them, liberals want to use it to compel people to do what's good for them, and psychiatrists want to use it to compel them to do both. This is why psychiatry is embraced by conservatives and liberals alike; why some libertarians ignore or tacitly support its coercive practices; and why most people view psychiatry not as therapeutic despotism but as the diagnosis and treatment of genuine diseases.

Liberty and Insanity

Justice is defined by custom and ratified by law. This is what makes it possible, morally and linguistically, to speak of "unjust laws," and gives force to utterances such as Camus's famous *cri de coeur:* "On the day when crime dons the apparel of innocence...it is innocence that is called upon to justify itself."[17] Today, many people who regard themselves as freedom-loving condone psychiatric violence clothed in the apparel of benevolence, and view the psychiatrist as a caring physician who restores the victims of mental illness to true freedom.

The American Civil Liberties Union, the country's premier civil liberties organization, supports depriving innocent persons of liberty, and persons accused of crimes of responsibility, provided psychiatrists diagnose the subjects as "mentally ill and dangerous."[18]

Leading libertarian organizations avoid making this mistake. Their failure—the Libertarian Party happily excepted—is the sin of silence, not condemning psychiatric deprivations of liberty and responsibility. The web site of the Institute for Justice—which identifies itself as "the nation's premier libertarian public interest law firm"—states:

> We are in courts across the country preserving freedom of opportunity and challenging government's control over individuals' lives. We sue governments when they stand in the way of entrepreneurs who seek to earn an honest living free from arbitrary and oppressive government interference. We litigate on behalf of individuals whose private property rights are threatened by government excesses. We represent parents who seek to choose the education that best meets their children's needs. We defend individuals' rights to publish and access information regardless of the communications medium involved. ... Our cases demonstrate that individual initiative, freedom of enterprise, freedom of speech, private property rights, and the legal protection of these liberties are vital to the future of all Americans....[19]

I applaud the Institute's work. I note here, with regret, only that its understanding of "challenging government's control over individuals' lives" does not encompass contesting what may well be the government's *most common and most insidious control over the lives of individuals—control by means of psychiatry.*

The best-known and most influential libertarian organization in the United States is the Cato Institute. Its web site states:

> [The Cato Institute] is a non-profit public policy research foundation...named for Cato's Letters, a series of libertarian pamphlets that helped lay the philosophical foundation for the American Revolution.... We reject the bashing of gays, Japan, rich people, and immigrants that contemporary liberals and conservatives seem to think addresses society's problems. We applaud the liberation of blacks and women from the statist restrictions that for so long kept them out of the economic mainstream. Our greatest challenge today is to extend the promise of political freedom and economic opportunity to those who are still denied it, in our own country and around the world.[20]

The Cato Institute, like the Institute for Justice, tends to equate individual liberty with economic liberty. Again, I applaud the Cato Institute's contributions to promoting a free society and note, with regret, that its publications dwell on the separation of the economy and the state, and pass over in silence about the union of psychiatry and the state.

For libertarians who take both their credo and the true social function of psychiatry seriously, the brightest star in the heavens is the Libertarian Party, "America's largest and most successful third party."[21] The Party's 2002 National Platform declares, *inter alia*: "We oppose the involuntary commitment of any person to, or involuntary treatment in, a mental institution.... We favor an end to the acceptance of criminal defenses based on 'insanity' or 'diminished capacity' which absolve the guilty of their responsibility."[22]

From Irresponsible Ward to Responsible Adult

Protestantism and the Enlightenment mark the beginnings of Western man's efforts to reject his status as the ward of God. The classic Greco-Roman ideal of freedom as personal independence is reborn. Man begins the long, hard struggle to grow up—to control his animal appetites, plan his own projects, and assume responsibility for the consequences of his actions.

Protestantism in effect limits the Christian God to mind his own business: It ordains men to take responsibility for their lives and be rewarded or punished for what they do with it. Enlightenment philosophy similarly limits the sovereign, the state, to mind its business, defined as protecting and promoting the "public good," leaving men at liberty to conduct their private lives within the bounds of the law and their own conscience.

Many men have offered perceptive remarks about modern, secular man's quest to free himself from his ostensibly protected, but actually oppressed, status as the ward of God. James Madison minced no words. "Religious bondage," he declared, "shackles and debilitates the mind and unfits it for every noble enterprise."[23]

What should be our standard for judging an enterprise or a project noble? I agree with Camus's criterion: "[T]he aim of life can only be to increase the sum of freedom and responsibility to be found in every man and in the world. It cannot, under any circumstances, be to reduce or suppress that freedom, even temporarily."[24] This goal is accessible to everyone, regardless of his station in life.

No one is born with a project. Everyone must develop one for himself. Toiling to support one's self and family—the project most people
in the world are saddled with—can be as noble as trying to unravel the
mysteries of nature or endeavoring to govern men with justice and wisdom. The quest is noble so long as it enlarges the sphere of liberty and
responsibility—for a single person, a family, or a multitude. It is ignoble
in proportion as it seeks, however "benevolently," to do otherwise. Basically, this is the libertarian project (whose death "end-of-history"-Francis
Fukuyama gleefully celebrates[25]).

I venture to say that, properly understood, libertarianism is as much
about responsibility as it is about liberty. Famously, Edmund Burke remarked: "Society cannot exist unless a controlling power upon will and
appetite be placed somewhere, and the less there is within, the more there
must be without."[26] Lord Acton rearticulated this "law of self-government" in slightly different terms: "Liberty is the prevention of control by
others. This requires self-control and, therefore, religious and spiritual
influences; education, knowledge, well-being."[27] In proportion as we
control our behavior and abstain from violating the rights of others, we
are entitled to enjoy the fruits of liberty.

This noble edifice is fatally undermined by the fiction of mental illness.
We claim that mental illness is the name of a bodily disease, but use it to
identify behaviors and "conditions" for which we do not hold the actor
responsible, because this fictitious illness supposedly impairs his ability
to control himself. This notion entails the additional belief that a "victim
of mental illness" is, at least temporarily, not fit for liberty, and must be
"treated" for his illness to make him fit again. This package of ideas and
interventions must be seen for what it is—a modern, humanistic-scientis-
tic dehumanization of man.[28] I have written extensively about this subject
elsewhere.[29] Two recent examples should suffice here.

- After being discharged from a mental hospital, Kevin Presland, an involuntarily hospitalized patient, stabs to death his prospective sister-in-law,
  Kelley-Anne Laws. He is acquitted of the crime on the ground of insanity,
  is confined for two years and sues the hospital for having released him prematurely. The court awards him $300,000 in damages. The judge explains,
  "that while it was generally unacceptable for someone to recover damages
  where they had committed a crime, in this case 'he was insane at the time
  of the killing and innocent of any crime.'" Presland admitted that in the days
  before he killed Laws, "he drank up to 10 schooners of beer and smoked six
  doses of marijuana daily, which the court heard precipitated his psychosis.
  Police took him to *hospital* after an altercation at a friend's house, where
  he had tried to strangle a child, and thought his friend was "in league with

the devil." Christine Laws, the victim's mother, "was devastated at yester-day's judgement. 'Don't give it to him, [she said]. It was his choice to take marijuana, his choice to drink—nobody else's. No one made him do it, yet the system sees fit to pay him. I can't understand the law.'"[30]

* "After threatening to take his own life and harm his mother," Joshua Daniel Lee is committed for a three-day psychiatric observation. On January 7, 2001, he is released. On January 29, he attacks and stabs to death Diane S. Bragg. One week later, he hangs himself in his jail cell. Bragg's adult sons sue the psychiatrists who had treated their father. The psychiatrists petition the court for dismissal on the ground that they had no "duty to warn" Diane Bragg, as Lee had never told them he planned to harm her. A three-panel California Appeals Court upheld the right of the plaintiffs to sue."[31]

In a free society, an adult can be coerced only for the benefit of so-ciety—by the police, if he is suspected of a crime, and by the judge, if he is convicted of one. In such a society, an adult is not supposed to be coerced for his own benefit—by educational authorities, to improve his mind; by religious authorities, to save his soul; or by medical authori-ties, to protect his health. Yet, he can be and is coerced by psychiatric authorities, to treat his mental illness.

The libertarian premise that people are responsible for their actions, and the psychiatric premise that mental illness diminishes or annuls re-sponsibility, are mutually incompatible. Libertarians must either subscribe to the mythology of mental illness and the use of violence it justifies, or reject the psychiatric creed and repudiate the deprivations of liberty it justifies. Psychiatric slavery—like chattel slavery—is an either/or issue.[32] A person either supports it or opposes it. *Tertium non datur.*

I

Principles:

Why Libertarianism and Psychiatry are Incompatible

1

Responsibility:
The Moral Foundation of Liberty

Incarceration in prisons and mental hospitals are clear instances of deprivation of liberty. The former is justified by the prisoner's guilt, the latter by the patient's mental illness. Crime implies injury to the life, liberty, or property of others. Mental illness implies "dangerousness" to self or others and non-responsibility for one's (mis)behavior. These truisms frame the context for my criticism of many libertarians' acceptance of the concept of mental illness, which constitutes the vital center of the ideology of mental health.

No term in the English language today expresses the idea that certain persons are not fit for liberty and are not responsible for their illegal actions more powerfully than does the term "mental illness." The term "mental illness" is virtually synonymous with nonresponsibility. Our everyday language expresses this organic connection: people excuse others and themselves of responsibility for misbehavior by calling the actor not only "mentally ill" but also "crazy," "delusional," "insane," "nuts," "schizophrenic," "psychotic," "not himself," "out of his mind," and so forth.[1] The insanity defense—which requires a diagnosis of mental illness by accredited psychiatrists and psychologists—epitomizes this magical-religious role of the idea of mental illness in the administration of the criminal law.[2]

To ignore this moral and legal aspect of the concept of mental illness is like ignoring the proverbial elephant in the room. For more than three centuries, experts on the mind—mad doctors, alienists, psychiatrists, and psychologists—have clung to the idea of mental illness like a drowning man clings to a raft. It is understandable that they do so. As the identity and prestige of the priest depend on the existence of God, so the identity and prestige of the psychiatrist and clinical psychologist depend on the existence of mental illness. It does not matter how God or mental illness is defined. What matters is that their existence or reality be accepted.

3

Freedom and Independence

In the English-speaking world, the word "freedom" has long been synonymous with the right to life, liberty, and property, the first two elements resting on the last. More than any other single principle, this idea informed and animated the Framers of the Constitution. "If the United States mean to obtain and deserve the full praise due to wise and just governments," wrote James Madison in 1792, "they will equally respect the rights of property and the property in rights."[3]

The essential feature of capitalism, as a political-economic system, is the security of private property. To ensure a free social order, the state must protect people from force and fraud by criminals at home and enemies abroad, and abstain from participating in the production and distribution of goods and services. Of course, no such perfect capitalist order, protected by a minimalist state, has ever existed or, perhaps, could exist. Inexorably, the protector is corrupted by his power. Nor can we ignore the intense human need for security—provided by religion or state—as an ever-present counterweight to the human need for liberty. This is the context that frames the contemporary interest in, and importance of, libertarianism as a secular religion and political force, much as the colonial status of Americans in the mid-eighteenth century framed the context for the Declaration of Independence.

The Declaration of Independence is the document the Founders used to justify the Colonies' secession from the English Crown, and for claiming their rightful place as the United States at the table of sovereign nations. It is a proclamation by a collectivity—a group of people defined primarily by geography—of its independence as a nation. National independence, however, is not personal independence. Nationalism is not individualism.

Libertarianism as a Declaration of Personal Independence complements Americanism, embodied in the Declaration of Independence as a proclamation of national independence. It is an affirmation of autonomy and self-responsibility and a rejection of the coercive paternalism of the modern state. Libertarianism—as the "Religion" of Personal Liberty and Responsibility—needs a formal Declaration of Independence. I propose the following preamble for it.

DECLARATION OF LIBERTARIAN-RESPONSIBILITARIAN INDEPENDENCE:

We hold these truths to be self-evident: that all men are created equal, and that the dignity inherent in their manhood entails that they be held responsible for their actions by themselves as well as by others. Their Creator has, accordingly, endowed them with inalienable Responsibility—that is, account-ability for their actions; this obligation cannot be denied them by others, nor can it be rejected by them. Foremost among man's obligations are the responsibility to assume ownership over himself; respect the personhood and rights of others; support himself and those who, by his freely chosen actions, are dependent on him, and, to this end, cooperate with others; and eschew initiating violence against others, particularly in what may appear to be the others' interest.

The Primacy of Responsibility

Historically as well as morally, responsibility is anterior to liberty. Children have, or ought to have, responsibilities before they have liber-ties. This does not contradict the view, to which I adhere, that liberty and responsibility go hand in hand, that they are two sides of the same moral coin. It's a case of which comes first, the chicken or the egg, and I suggest that we treat the chicken as if it does. Individuals and groups cannot be free if they are unwilling to restrain their inclinations to deprive others of the freedom they want for themselves: their primary duty is to govern themselves, not others.

We are controlled, and control others, by punishments and rewards, the stick and the carrot. The Bill of Rights offers us certain protections from the state's use of the stick—its apparatus of coercion. Unfortunately, it does not safeguard us from the state's use of the carrot—"rights to" education, health care, welfare, and other "benefits." This is the famil-iar danger posed by redistributionist-socialist policies. Fifty years ago, conservative writer Garet Garrett observed: "In these twenty years, a revolution took place in the relationship between government and people. Formerly government was the responsibility of people; now people are the responsibility of government."[4] If people are the responsibility of government, it is the duty of the state to provide them with safety nets, protecting them from poverty, disease, and, perhaps most importantly, *from themselves*. Hence the therapeutic state and its myriad rules and laws regulating drugs, gambling, sex, suicide, and mental illness.

What is wrong with such a polity? It provides for human needs that independent adults, who want to be free, ought to provide for themselves. If they let the state make available to them benefits they could supply for themselves—such as employment, education for their children, informa-tion about what foods to eat and drugs to take—they will, like it or not, become infantilized and grow increasingly dependent on the state. They will begin to define and treat themselves and others not as responsible agents but as victims of poverty, discrimination, drug abuse, child abuse, and mental illness. This is the tragedy of our present condition: "rights" that are really regulations, such as the right to medical care or welfare, multiply, yet at the same time we are deprived of genuine rights, such as the rights to self-medication and suicide.[5] In a social order based on and honoring the rule of law and the free market, adults must have the right to be wrong, no less than the right to be right. I suggest that we categorize the right to be "mentally ill" as an instance of the right to be wrong. (If the person said to be mentally ill deprives others of their right to life, liberty, and property, he ought to be treated the same way as we treat persons not said to be mentally ill who commit such crimes.)

A brief look at the language of psychiatry is, as always, instructive. Fifty years ago, psychiatrists spoke about mental illness and mental disease, neurosis and psychosis. Today, they use these terms less frequently. Instead, psychiatrists speak about "mental disorder," a term that further discredits their medical claims. When I was young, psychiatrists acknowledged that neurotics were *disturbed*, and psychotics were *disturbing*. Now they claim that all such persons have "disorders." Persons called "mental patients" are either *disordered* (dissatisfied with themselves), or *disordering* (displeasing others). Revealingly, the term "disorderly conduct" refers to a type of criminal offense. However, most so-called mental disorders do not name acts that constitute crimes and are therefore not punishable by criminal penalties. Instead, they constitute offenses against mental health laws and are punishable by psychiatric "treatments."

Libertarians rightly point out that the free market "works" better than does the command economy. Precisely therein lies the reason why many libertarians are reluctant to oppose psychiatry.

Since the seventeenth century, it has become increasingly clear that free labor is more economically productive than slave labor, and that cooperation and contract are morally preferable to domination and coercion. Since the fall of the Soviet empire, few people doubt that a market economy based on contract offers a more effective means for raising peoples' material well being than does a command economy based on force. This leads to the obvious question: If market relations are such an effective method for protecting us from material discomfort and suffering, why have such relations not become the universal means of conducting human affairs? Adam Smith answered: "To expect...that the freedom of trade should ever be entirely restored in Great Britain, is as absurd as to expect that an Oceana or Utopia should ever be established in it. Not only the prejudices of the public, but what is much more unconquerable, the private interests of many individuals, irresistibly oppose it."[6] Smith was too optimistic. He assumed that people want peace and prosperity to pursue their private, productive activities, working, marrying, raising children.

Standing on the shoulders of Adam Smith and the Austrian economists, we can offer a more comprehensive answer. Many human relations—notably, those between parents and children, family members, and friends—fall outside the scope of exchange and reciprocity, strictly defined. All human relations entail some form or measure of reciprocity, even relations between oppressor and oppressed. However, the reciprocity that characterizes arm's-length business relations governed by contract and enforceable by law is very different from the reciprocity that characterizes intimate relations between people bound to one another by affectional, as opposed to legal, ties. Some of these relationships require a measure of coercion. Others require a recognition of the legitimacy of domination and submission. Libertarian principles are not an existential panacea: they do not cure every ailment of the human condition. I am not implying that libertarians make such a claim. Indeed, this mistake is typically made by critics of libertarianism. The libertarian philosophy of liberty ought to be seen as a lodestar pointing the way to the development of the free human spirit in the atmosphere of a free society. That is enough of an achievement.

With respect to psychiatry, the challenge to libertarians is not to be blinded by the slogan "it works."[7] In certain aspects of life—in religion, politics, and psychiatry—*everything works, and nothing works.* The value of libertarianism as an ethic is not that "it works," but that it promotes liberty and responsibility. Stupidity does not work. Laziness does not work. Poor personal hygiene does not work. But we, libertarians, oppose agents of the state interfering in the lives of persons on such grounds. We do so not because we value stupidity, laziness, or poor personal hygiene, but because we value freedom.

The behaviors we call "mental illnesses" both work and do not work. Some work perfectly well for the subject: they are habits or patterns of behavior that satisfy his needs and values—but dissatisfy others, especially members of his family. At the same time, most such behaviors do not work, in the sense that they do not help make the subject healthy, wealthy, happy, or virtuous. Regardless of these considerations, people should have a *right to be "mentally ill" or "mentally disordered,"* just as they have a right to be personally disordered. Of course, people we so label or who so label themselves should not be excused for their law-breaking on the ground of fictitious mental disorders.

Similarly, the coercions we call "psychiatric treatments" may also be said to both work and not work. They work in the sense that they satisfy the needs of family members and society by the disposing of persons who disturb them and by disguising their removal as medical treatment. On the other hand, they obviously do not work: they do not relieve or cure "mental illnesses" or the idleness, indigence, and crime we associate with such "diseases."

We do not ask, Does religion work? We acknowledge that persons who practice their religion believe it works (and the other way around). The point is that we regard the voluntary practice of religion as a basic human right, and prohibit its involuntary practice as a criminal act. Our attitude toward psychiatry ought to be the same. Instead of asking whether psychiatry works, we ought to acknowledge that it does if the patient contracts and pays for it (and the other way around); protect the practice of voluntary psychiatry, *de facto* prohibited by the therapeutic state, as a basic human right;[8] and insist that the practice of involuntary psychiatry be prohibited as a crime against humanity.[9] Libertarians tend to overlook that psychiatry is a socialist-statist institution, similar to a state religion, such as Catholicism in medieval times or Islam in Saudi Arabia today. Psychiatry, like religion, provides rules and regulations for personal and social conduct, not diagnoses and treatments for bodily illnesses. Traditionally, religion and the state formed one institution and all three monotheistic religions relied on coercion. In the West, they are now separate institutions, with religion dispossessed of the legitimate use of force.

In the United States today, psychiatry is united with the state the same way that religion and the state were formerly united virtually everywhere. If all mental health laws were repealed and the government were prohibited from funding psychiatric activities, psychiatry as we know it would cease to exist. The vacuum would, in all likelihood, be filled by many diverse and perhaps novel forms of "free" (contractual, noncoercive) psychiatry, helping services provided by philanthropic foundations and institutions, and, for lawbreakers, by criminal sanctions.

Have Economists Hijacked the Idea of Liberty?

Historically, the idea of freedom rests primarily on a moral and philosophical basis. Montesquieu, Voltaire, and Zola in France; Adam Smith, Mill, and Acton in England; Franklin, Jefferson, and Paine in America—none of these men based the case for liberty on economic arguments. I am not gainsaying the crucial importance for individual liberty of the right to property and a rule of law protecting that right. I am merely saying that liberty is not the sole "possession" of free-market economists. Recently, Llewellyn H. Rockwell, Jr. cogently argued that the very economic superiority of the market over the socialist system of production is a danger to liberty. He observed:

> Among the greatest failures of the free-market intellectual movement has been to allow its ideas to be categorized as a "public policy" option. The formulation implies...that the purpose of freedom, private ownership, and market incentives is the superior management of society.... There are many examples of this awful concession operating today. In policy circles, people use the word privatization to mean not the bowing out of government from a particular aspect of social and economic life, but merely the contracting out of statist priorities to politically connected private enterprise. School vouchers and Social Security "privatization" are the most notorious examples at the national level.... What's at stake is the very conception of the role of freedom in political, economic, and social life.... The worst mistake our side can make is to sell our ideas as a better means for achieving the state's ends. *Yet this approach—advertising market economics as the best political option among a variety of plans—has become the dominant one on our side of the fence....* Freedom is not a public-policy option. It is the end of public policy itself.[10]

I would go a little farther. By overemphasizing the relations between freedom and the free market, economists have hijacked the idea of liberty. They have made it appear as if individual liberty were a consequence or by-product of the market and of the economic growth and material prosperity it promotes. This is a fundamental fallacy. Material prosperity neither guarantees freedom nor is a measure of it. *Indeed, operating in a basically statist framework, the market economy is a danger to freedom.*

After spending nearly a century pitting Austrian economics against Marxism, Keynesianism, and Communism, libertarians have become accustomed to defending liberty on economic grounds, that is, demonstrating that a market economy makes people better off in terms of material well being than does a socialist economy. But, obviously, it also makes the state better off. Herein lies what, following Hayek, we might call the "fatal conceit" of libertarianism.[11]

It is precisely because the market economy enriches the state more than does the command economy that the United States won the arms race and the Cold War. It is also why our daily lives are increasingly constrained and suffocated by the deadly embrace of a therapeutic state.

2

The Libertarian Credo and the Ideology of Psychiatry

"That government is best which governs least" is the maxim with which Henry David Thoreau (1817-1862) opens his pamphlet, *Civil Disobedience* (1849).[1] This statement, often erroneously attributed to Thomas Jefferson, sums up the nineteenth-century, classical liberal concept of good government.[2] The term "liberalism" then denoted the political philosophy of minimal government, its scope and powers limited by the rule of law. Individuals flourished—minding their own business and cooperating with others as need be—when left alone by agents of the state. Viewing the state as possessing a monopoly on the legally justified use of force, the nineteenth-century liberal saw it as a threat to individual liberty.

In the eighteenth century, there also came into being a very different concept of political philosophy, later called "utilitarianism." In 1725, the Irish-English philosopher Francis Hutcheson (1694-1746) articulated the formula destined for fame: "That Action is best which procures the greatest Happiness for the greatest Numbers; and that worst, which, in like manner, occasions misery."[3] Although Hutcheson used the term "Action" to refer to personal conduct, not government policy, the principle he annunciated became the foundation of a system of anti-individualistic political philosophy that Jeremy Bentham (1748-1832) named "utilitarianism."[4]

The Scottish philosopher David Hume (1711-1776) reformulated Hutcheson's statement as an explicitly political principle. He wrote: "The good and happiness of the members, that is the majority of the members of the state, is the great standard by which every thing relating to that state must finally be determined."[5] In the nineteenth century, his libertarian leanings notwithstanding, John Stuart Mill's (1806-1873) book on utilitarianism gave a big impetus to this collectivistic political philosophy.[6] In this view, the state is an organ of benevolence, providing people with

11

the goods and services they need. The greater the scope of government, the better it can assist and protect the welfare of the people.

In the Declaration of Independence, as a compromise over slavery, the Founders replaced the phrase "right to property" with the phrase "right to the pursuit of happiness." This was very unfortunate. To be sure, they expected people to pursue happiness on their own behalf, not have the government provide them with it. Still, the term "happiness" in the Declaration resonates perilously with the utilitarian-political principle of "greatest happiness." That standard, as Lord Acton warned, is inimical to liberty: "If happiness is the end of society, then liberty is superfluous. It does not make men happy."[7]

As the nineteenth century turned into the twentieth, the terms "liberal" and "utilitarian" that denoted these opposing philosophies of governance began to change. Persons who formerly called themselves liberals now call themselves libertarians or classical liberals (or sometimes conservatives), while their opponents call them reactionaries or right-wingers. Persons who formerly called themselves utilitarians now call themselves "liberals" and "progressives," while their opponents call them "socialists" and "statists." In the early days of the twentieth century, in the United States, the new liberal tended to be virtually synonymous with the Democrat, and the classical liberal synonymous with the Republican. After the Second World War, however, Democrats and Republicans alike became advocates of Big Government, each seeking to use the coercive power of the state to impose its "moral vision" on the people. This drift towards statism by both left and right lent impetus to the formation and growth of contemporary libertarianism.

As is often the case with terms that are used more to praise or condemn than to describe or identify, the dictionary definitions of the term "libertarian" are singularly unhelpful. *Webster's* defines libertarian as "advocating a theory of free will; advocating or advancing liberty"; and libertarianism as "the theories or practices of a libertarian." *The Oxford English Dictionary* states: "Libertarian: one who holds the doctrine of the freedom of the will, as opposed to that of necessity; one who approves of or advocates liberty."

The credit for giving the term its present meaning belongs to Dean Russell, one of the founders of the Foundation for Economic Education (FEE). In 1955, he stated: "Strictly speaking, a libertarian is one who rejects the idea of using violence or the threat of violence—legal or illegal—to impose his will or viewpoint upon any peaceful person. Generally speaking, a libertarian is one who wants to be governed far less than he is today."[8] This is an elegant identification of one of the core principles of libertarianism, namely, the essential wrongfulness of using violence "to do good." However, Russell's definition is silent about another, closely related core principle, namely, that adults own themselves and hence should, *a priori*, be free of arbitrary government interference. This principle is a reformulation of the moral ground for the Declaration of Independence: "We hold these truths to be self-evident, that all men are created equal; that they are endowed by their Creator with inherent and inalienable rights; that among these, are life, liberty, and the pursuit of happiness..."

The Principle of Nonaggression

The father of the principle of not initiating violence, also called the principle of nonaggression, is John Locke. In his *Second Treatise of Government* (1690), he stated:

> [T]here being nothing more evident than that creatures of the same species and rank promiscuously born to all the same advantages of nature and use of the same faculties, should also be equal amongst another without subordination of subjection.... The state of nature has a law of nature to govern it which obliges every one; and reason, which is that law, teaches all mankind who will consult it that, being all equal and independent, *no one ought to harm another in his life, health, liberty, or possessions....*[9]

This prescription is, in effect, synonymous with the prescription that, as human beings, we have an "inalienable" right to life, liberty, and property. There is general agreement among libertarians that this precept is the bedrock principle of the philosophy of libertarianism. Murray Rothbard put it thus:

> The libertarian creed rests upon one central axiom: that no man or group of men may aggress against the person or property of anyone else. This may be called the "nonaggression axiom." "Aggression" is defined as the initiation of the use or threat of physical violence against the person or property of anyone else. Aggression is therefore synonymous with invasion...this at once implies that the libertarian stands foursquare for what are generally known as "civil liberties": the freedom to speak, publish, assemble, and engage in such "victimless crimes" as pornography, sexual deviation, and prostitution....[10]

Walter Block reiterates this principle: "The foundation of libertarianism is the non-aggression axiom. This states that it is illicit to initiate or threaten invasive violence against a man or his legitimately owned property. Murray Rothbard characterized this as 'plumb line' libertarianism: follow this one principle, and you will be able to infer the libertarian position on all issues, without exception."[11]

Reconciling the foundational libertarian principle of not initiating aggression with the fundamental psychiatric practice of initiating the use of force or threatening its initiation against persons denominated as mental patients poses a problem most libertarians are not eager to confront. Murray Rothbard was an exception. He stated:

> One of the most shameful areas of involuntary servitude in our society is the widespread practice of compulsory commitment, or involuntary hospitalization, of mental patients. In former generations this incarceration of noncriminals was frankly carried out as a measure against mental patients, to remove them from society. The practice of twentieth-century liberalism has been superficially more humane, but actually far more insidious: now physicians and psychiatrists help incarcerate these unfortunates "for their own good." The humanitarian rhetoric has permitted a far more widespread use of the practice and, for one thing, has allowed disgruntled relatives to put away their loved ones without suffering a guilty conscience.[12]

As I noted in the Introduction, the Libertarian Party's Platform takes seriously that libertarian ideas must have libertarian consequences, not only with respect to the market in housing and plumbing services, but also with respect to what we euphemistically call "mental health services." I reproduce below the part of the Platform especially relevant to our present concerns:

> We believe that respect for individual rights is the essential precondition for a free and prosperous world, that force and fraud must be banished from human relationships, and that only through freedom can peace and prosperity be realized. Consequently, we defend each person's right to engage in any activity that is peaceful and honest, and welcome the diversity that freedom brings....
>
> We hold that all individuals have the right to exercise sole dominion over their own lives, and have the right to live in whatever manner they choose, so long as they do not forcibly interfere with the equal right of others to live in whatever manner they choose.... Since governments, when instituted, must not violate individual rights, we oppose all interference by government in the areas of voluntary and contractual relations among individuals....
>
> Victimless Crimes: Because only actions that infringe on the rights of others can properly be termed crimes, we favor the repeal of all federal, state, and local laws creating "crimes" without victims. In particular, we advocate:
> [T]he repeal of all laws prohibiting the production, sale, possession, or use of drugs, and of all medicinal prescription requirements for the purchase of vitamins, drugs, and similar substances;...
> Health Care: ...We advocate a complete separation of medicine and State....

Government and Mental Health: We oppose the involuntary commitment of any person to or involuntary treatment in a mental institution. We strongly condemn Involuntary Outpatient Commitment (IOC), where the patient is ordered to accept treatment, or else be committed to a mental institution and forcibly treated. We oppose government pressure requiring parents to obtain counseling or psychiatric drugs for their children. We also oppose forced treatment for the elderly, the head-injured, or those with diminished capacity. Medication must be voluntary. We are against the invasion of people's homes and privacy by health officials or law enforcement to either require or deny drug taking. We advocate an end to the spending of tax money for any program of psychiatric, psychological, or behavioral research or treatment. We favor an end to the acceptance of criminal defenses based on "insanity" or "diminished capacity" which absolve the guilty of their responsibility.[13]

It is difficult for me to see how a person who espouses the "libertarian theology of freedom" (Edmund A. Opitz's term) could settle for anything less.[14] Still, many civil libertarians and libertarians support the psychiatric enterprise, either explicitly or by their silence. The American Civil Liberties Union, as I show later, is in effect a mouthpiece of the American Psychiatric Association. Many libertarians, for their part, dwell on the importance of free markets, except in psychiatry, and tirelessly recite the mantra that "people should be free to do whatever they want in life as long as their conduct is peaceful," but do not mention mental health laws, much less advocate their repeal. For example, Charles Murray, the Bradley Fellow at the American Enterprise Institute (AEI) and the author of several acclaimed libertarian tracts on social policy, states: "Applied to personal behavior, the libertarian ethic is simple but stark: Thou shalt not initiate the use of force."[15] Yet, in his book, *What It Means to Be a Libertarian*, he does not mention psychiatry, let alone its unyielding commitment to initiating the use of force.[16]

Psychiatry and the Problem of What Counts as Initiating Violence

The language we use to describe human relations is rarely value neutral. The libertarian term "initiating violence" is pejorative: it implies an action we ought to avoid. Conversely, the psychiatric term "treatment" is commendatory: it implies an action we ought to perform. The crux of the problem is that an act that, from a libertarian point of view, is coercive is, from a psychiatric point of view, therapeutic. Let us see if we can throw light, as well as some heat, on this problem.

Dictionary definitions of key terms afford a convenient beginning, but no more than that. *Webster's* defines aggression as "a culpable, unprovoked, overt hostile attack...violating rights"; violence as "the exertion of any physical force so as to injure or abuse"; and initiate as "to begin or set going." These bare bones need a great deal of fleshing out. Missing here is reference to self-ownership, the body, and consent. Many of the most glaring acts of violence in and among modern states are avowedly committed to "help" or "liberate" the assaulted people or nation, and hence do not fit the definition of violence as "the exertion of any physical force so as to injure or abuse."

Let us start with a simple case. A young woman starves herself. Her parents turn for help to a psychiatrist. He diagnoses the woman, henceforth called a "patient," as suffering from anorexia nervosa, incarcerates and forcibly feeds her. The woman regards these acts as unjustified violence. Her family, psychiatrists, society, and the law regard them as life-saving treatment.

This example highlights the crucial importance of not losing sight of our instinctive belief that *our bodies are our property, they belong to us*. This is why it is a fundamental legal principle that any unauthorized penetration or even unwanted touching of the body constitutes a criminal offense. Except in emergencies—about which more in a moment—medical treatment without consent constitutes assault and battery, regardless of whether it medically benefits the subject. The prohibition against violating the body extends even past death: we have far-reaching rights over determining what happens to our corpse.

There are two major exceptions to the general principle of the sanctity of the body we must now consider. One is the relationship of parent to minor child, the other is the relationship between physician and patient.

By virtue of biological necessity, parents have certain rights to invade the bodies of their minor children. Children do not consent to being conceived and brought into the world. The very process of birth is an act of violence on the baby. During early infancy, the parent must assume a degree of control over the child's bodily functions. That control, however, is far from complete. Church and state also claim their share of control over the child. Throughout history, religion and law have set limits to parental power, especially with respect to life and sex: virtually all such codes prohibit the parent's killing the child or using the child's body as a means for the parent's sexual gratification.

Medicine and Violence

The medical professional's relationship to the human body is more subtle and more complex. This is the main source of confusion about precisely what, in a psychiatric context, counts as "initiating violence"—a confusion that infects even many libertarian minds. I noted that our life begins in what surely looks like an act of violence. Women used to talk about being "torn apart" in the process of childbirth. In the modern world, most people are shielded from the event. Those who witness it often faint at its bloody violence. And that is but the beginning of the deep-seated connections between medicine and violence.

A great deal of the practice of medicine takes place at three paradigmatic "scenes of violence": the autopsy table, the operating room, and the emergency room. At the first scene, the dead body is dissected and parts of it are removed. At the second, the living human body is carved up. At the third, a seriously injured person is subjected to violent interventions. In each case, the physician engages in acts that, *outside of a medical context*, would constitute felonious assaults against the body and the person. Why do we not count these "aggressions" against the body as instances of violence? Because we accept the *conventional justifications* for them. The autopsy is justified by the consent of the patient or his next of kin, as well as on criminological, scientific, and educational grounds. Surgery and emergency treatment are justified by consent, explicit or implied. The result is that many physicians, accustomed to committing acts of sanctioned violence, fall into the habit of justifying coercion as care. Mixed with feelings of superiority and lack of accountability, compassion and morality are quickly blunted. To make matters worse, the new discipline of bioethics is devoted largely to rationalizing and legitimizing medically sanctioned violence, most obviously in psychiatry.

The judgment of all human acts is subject to the observer's values. What counts as a violent act? What counts as a sexual act? I offer a sardonic litmus test, inspired by the popularity of television: if it's on TV, it's either violence or sex or both. I submit that the attraction of television shows featuring emergency rooms lies mainly in their violence, which is typically two-fold: we see the victim hemorrhaging from a life-threatening wound and physicians resorting to "heroic" measures to save his life. Even if the medical problem is not the result of a criminal act, the scene is likely to be one of violence. The patient's arrival is heralded by the screaming sound of an ambulance; doctors and attendants run around in bloody attire; hysterical relatives crowd the hallways. The patient,

vomiting blood or unconscious, is assailed by medical personnel insert-
ing things into his mouth and veins. It is a tableau we typically describe
in military metaphors: the patient is "attacked" by disease; the doctors
"fight" to save him.

A small change in the scenario brings us to the heart of our problem.
The typical mental patient in the emergency room is the victim of neither
assault nor illness. Indeed, he is, strictly speaking, not a patient but a
prisoner. For example, a middle-aged, unhappily married man tells his
wife he is going to kill himself. She calls the police. Instead of coming to
the ER in an ambulance, the denominated patient arrives in handcuffs, in
a police van. Diagnosis: "Bipolar illness, psychotic depression; patient is
dangerous to himself and others." Treatment: Involuntary mental hospitalization and the forcible administration of an antipsychotic drug.

To be sure, calling such a person's treatment "imprisonment" is an
insult to the psychiatric profession. That is understandable. Psychiatry
is incompatible with liberty. *Black's Law Dictionary* states: "Every confinement of the person is an 'imprisonment,' whether it be in a common
prison, or in private house, or in the stocks, or even by forcibly detaining
one in the public streets."[17]

To the untrained, unskeptical mind—and especially to the psychiatrically "enlightened" mind—the psychiatric emergency and the surgical
emergency appear to be similar, even identical. Both cases are treated as
"medical emergencies"; both subjects are brought to emergency rooms
and given emergency medical treatment. What is the difference between
them? The answer lies in what, more than forty years ago, I called the
"myth of mental illness."[18] I shall articulate the differences as they apply
specifically to the emergency scenarios I have sketched.

•   In the case of the medical emergency, the subject suffers from a life-
     threatening bodily injury or illness likely to cause death unless treated
     without delay; the patient is too incapacitated to request medical help or
     give or reject consent to treatment. Consent to medical care is implied
     in the situation or is granted by a next of kin.

•   In the case of the psychiatric emergency, the subject suffers from no
     injury or illness at all. He is conscious and capable of requesting medical
     help. However, he explicitly rejects medical interference. He is brought
     to the hospital by force and is declared *de facto* incompetent by the
     physician's "dual diagnosis" of "mental illness" and "dangerousness."

Psychiatry and Dangerousness

When we consider the relationship between libertarianism and psychiatry, it is necessary to keep in mind that mental health laws authorize, in effect compel, psychiatrists to deprive of liberty persons whom they regard as having a *mental illness* and posing a *danger* to themselves or others. Commitment laws do not require that the "patient" be, or be declared, mentally or legally *incompetent.* The psychiatrist's oracular declaration that the subject is "mentally ill" and "dangerous to himself and others" is enough to justify his incarceration. Consider this hypothetical scenario.

Over a period of weeks, a sniper shoots and kills several people. The police identify, arrest, and incarcerate him. *We regard the sniper, not the police, as having initiated violence.* The sniper, however, may insist that he did *not initiate violence, but that he was merely retaliating against unjust acts of violence against "his" people.*

Since the 1950s, this is exactly the sort of mutual accusation of initiating aggression that we have witnessed on the world stage, especially in the Middle East. Virtually every act of war and bloodshed has been justified by both parties as acts of morally justified *self-defense.* Typically, politicians have also justified the resort to violence as a measure intended to prevent or remedy an *emergency*, posed by enemies abroad or criminals or "dangerous diseases" at home. The emergency of the Civil War enabled Lincoln to transform the United States from a constitutional Republic into a centralized nation. Similarly, the emergencies of the Depression and World War II enabled Roosevelt to transform United States into a bureaucratic, regulatory, welfare state. "Every collective revolution," warned Herbert Hoover (1874-1964), "rides in on a Trojan horse of 'Emergency.' It was the tactic of Lenin, Hitler, and Mussolini.... This technique of creating emergency is the greatest achievement that demagoguery attains."[19] The infamous George Jacques Danton (1759-1794) declared: "Everything belongs to the fatherland when the fatherland is in danger."[20]

When this rationalization is advanced in a political context, libertarians see through it and reject it. However, when the same rationalization appears in a psychiatric context, libertarians are often taken in. They accept that the psychiatrist's pronouncing a person "mentally ill and dangerous" is a valid justification for initiating violence against him. In other words, they regard so-called psychiatric emergencies as instances of genuine medical emergencies.

One reason for this gullibility may be due to the power of unexamined words. Terms such as "crazy," "mentally ill," "mad," "schizophrenic," "suicidal," and "psychotic" connote and entail the idea of violence, that is, of an actor who has committed, or is about to commit, a violent act. Then, in a classic example of circular reasoning, when such a person commits a violent act, people accept the psychiatric interpretation that he did so because of his mental illness, that his illness "compelled" him to break the law, or to take his own life, an act that is *not against the criminal law.* In short, some libertarians uncritically accept the whole body of psychiatric diagnostics and the mental health laws used to enforce them.

Libertarians may also be uneasy about opposing *psychiatric violence*—the psychiatrist in effect arresting, judging, and imprisoning the mental patient—because they perceive the madman as being deluded and irrational, properly subject to care by more rational persons. Presently, I shall have more to say about the role of the terms "rational-irrational" in economics and psychiatry.[21] Here, a few preliminary remarks must suffice.

The person who makes a mistake—say, adding a series of numbers incorrectly—corrects it as soon as he discovers the error or it is pointed out to him. In contrast, the so-called psychotic person asserts his false claim—say, that he is Jesus Christ—and no evidence or argument will make him change his mind. I have suggested that many such false statements resemble religious beliefs and may be understood as metaphors, similar to a father calling his daughter, "My angel."[22] The point is that statements—regardless of whether they are true or false—are instances of *speech acts.* Making speech acts is a right protected by the First Amendment. Priests and politicians are permitted to assert what many believe are falsehoods. "Psychotics" are not. Psychiatrists deny the "severely ill" mental patient's right to prevaricate by "diagnosing" his falsehoods as "psychotic delusions." Clearly, speech acts of this type annoy and upset persons to whom they are addressed. As a rule, delusions are not threats and uttering them are not crimes. If we free ourselves from the grip of psychiatric convention, it is evident that asserting a falsehood about oneself or the world—"having" delusions and hallucinations—is not a crime. The person who asserts that he is God or has fifteen personalities is not an aggressor; he is a liar.

Nevertheless, psychiatrists routinely stigmatize persons who utter such falsehoods—epitomized by "hearing voices"—as "hallucinating" and "psychotic," and hence mentally ill and dangerous to themselves and others. Although such a determination may appear to be simply a medical judgment or opinion, in fact it is a legal determination. The psychiatrist who *certifies* that Jones is mentally ill and dangerous to himself and others is like a jury foreman who pronounces Jones guilty of a felony. The result is brutal injustice masquerading as benevolent treatment.

- The disposition to violence ("dangerousness") of the average felon serving jail time is evidenced by his past behavior. His punishment is a finite term of incarceration in prison.

- There is no objective evidence that the average severely ill mental patient has a disposition to violence ("dangerousness"). His treatment is an indefinite term of incarceration in a mental hospital.

From the point of view of a non-believer, claims about miracles and historic covenants with gods—the two paradigmatic manifestations of dogmatic faith—are falsehoods. One believer asserts that God commands him to circumcise his son, another that consecrated bread is the literal body of a resurrected man-god, a third that Allah is the one and only true god and that a man named Mohammed was his prophet.

Which of these assertions is true? Which is false? Which is a delusion? To stay out of that thicket, the libertarian advocates free religious speech and separation of church and state. To be consistent, he ought also to advocate free psychiatric speech and separation of psychiatry and the state. Surely, more violence has been committed, and continues to be committed, in the cause of religious claims than as a result of mental illnesses. I hazard the guess that the libertarian who is soft on psychiatry recoils from embracing the separation of psychiatry and the state because such a policy is now considered heretical—unaccepted and unacceptable by right-thinking persons.

The Principle of Self-Ownership

Some libertarians regard self-ownership as the movement's most basic principle, even more important than the principle of nonaggression. David Bergland—the Libertarian Party's presidential candidate in 1984—begins his book, *Libertarianism in One Lesson*, with this statement: "You Own Yourself.... No one else has the right to force you to act against your own interests as you see them."[23]

The self-ownership axiom obligates libertarians to oppose individuals and institutions that force us to act against our own interests. Bergland names only the usual libertarian suspects, such as drug prohibition, taxation, and state control of education. Psychiatry is conspicuous by its absence.

Bergland alludes to persons forced to act against their own interests. Who are these persons? To begin with, they are the classic trio of individuals who, in John Stuart Mill's terms, are of "nonage": infants, idiots, and the insane. There are also others: persons declared legally incompetent, diagnosed as mentally ill, imprisoned for crimes, having certain contagious diseases. For each class of coercible persons there is a class of individuals legally authorized to coerce them, for example, guardians, psychiatrists, jailers, and public health physicians. From the libertarian point of view, the powers of parents over children, jailers over prisoners, and legal guardians over wards is not nearly as important as are the powers of psychiatrists over mental patients.

The principle of self-ownership, unlike the principle of nonaggression, is deeply rooted in the concept of, and belief in, free will. This is what makes libertarians and some Christians bed-fellows. What else can the notion of free will mean other than "free will" over ourselves, our lives, our bodies? Surely, it cannot mean "free will" over the lives of others. "The free man," declared the great Christian humanist-humorist-philosopher Gilbert K. Chesterton in 1909, "owns himself. He can damage himself with either eating or drinking; he can ruin himself with gambling. If he does he is certainly a damn fool, and he might possibly be a damned soul; but if he may not, he is not a free man any more than a dog."[24] This is a far cry from the views of present-day Christian moral crusaders and anti-drug warriors, such as the infamous hypocrite, William Bennett.

In his perfectly titled book, *The Libertarian Theology of Freedom*, the Reverend Edmund A. Opitz—an ordained Congregational minister and a prominent "libertarian Christian"—bluntly states: "The business of society is peace; the business of government is violence. So, the question is: What service can violence render to peace? The libertarian answer is that violence can serve peace only by restraining peacebreakers."[25]

The Reverend Opitz rightly emphasizes that faith in freedom is a kind of religion and cites the great agnostic-skeptic, H. L. Mencken, to remind us that, "Of all the ideas associated with the general concept of democratic government, the oldest and perhaps the soundest is that of equality before the law. Its relation to the scheme of Christian ethics is too obvious to need statement. It goes back, through the political and theological theorizing of the middle ages, to the early Christian notion of equality before God.... The debt of democracy to Christianity has always been underestimated."[26]

I am in full agreement with this view and also with Opitz's comment: *"The freedom quest of Western man, as it has exhibited itself periodically over the past 20 centuries, is not a characteristic of man as such. It is a cultural trait, philosophically and religiously inspired."*[27]

In his Foreword to *The Libertarian Theology of Freedom*, Charles Hallberg, the publisher, perceptively states:

> In today's world, the term "libertarian Christian" seems to many people to be an oxymoron. It is not. It exemplifies nothing less than the true meaning of the teachings of Jesus.... Collectivism, under all its names—socialism, fascism, Nazism, communism and increasingly under the name of Democracy—derives its support from what Albert Jay Nock termed "Epstean's Law." That is, "Man tends always to satisfy his needs and desires with the least possible exertion." And what could be easier than using government to have someone else pay your bills? Or, for business to use government to limit competition and liability? Or, banking to gain a monopoly?[28]

We ought to add to Hallberg's examples a long list of "what could be easier" situations in which individuals, institutions, and the government use psychiatric interventions to resolve conflicts. For example, what could be easier than using government to help families rid themselves of annoying and embarrassing relatives? Or businesses, to discharge disruptive, "difficult" employees? Or schools, to use psychiatric drugs to incapacitate unruly children? Or courts, to declare defendants who threaten the social order but are not guilty of lawbreaking to be mentally ill and unfit to be tried and so avoid the trouble of putting them on trial? And so on.

Self-Ownership and the Courts

The United States Supreme Court is not usually thought of as a supporter of libertarian political principles. Nevertheless, it has repeatedly declared that, in American law, self-ownership is a "sacred" value. For example, in 1891, the Court stated: "No right is held more sacred, or is more carefully guarded by the common law, than the right of every individual to possession and control of his own person, free from all restraint or interference of others.... The right to one's person may be said to be a right of complete immunity: to be let alone."[29]

In 1928, Supreme Court Justice Louis D. Brandeis (1856-1941), a socialist, repeated that now-famous phrase and has since then been credited with it. He stated: "The makers of our Constitution sought to protect Americans in their beliefs, their thoughts, their emotions, and their sensations. They conferred, as against the Government, the right to be let alone—the most comprehensive of rights, and the right most valued by civilized men."[30]

In 1964, Chief Justice (then Circuit Judge) Warren Burger—in an often cited decision concerning the constitutionality of letting Jehovah's Witnesses reject life-saving blood transfusions—repeated Brandeis' admonition and added: "Nothing in this utterance suggests that Justice Brandeis thought an individual possessed these rights only as to *sensible* beliefs, *valid* thoughts, *reasonable* emotions, or *well-founded* sensations. I suggest he intended to include a great many foolish, unreasonable, and even absurd ideas which do not conform, such as refusing medical treatment even at great risk."[31]

A recent ruling by a court in California went so far as to interpret the right to be let alone as including the right to be let alone to commit suicide by self-starvation. In 1993, a prison physician sought a court order to permit him to use a surgical tube to feed and medicate a quadriplegic prisoner who had refused the intervention. The court ruled:

> Right to refuse medical treatment is equally "basic and fundamental" and integral to the concept of informed consent. Individual's right of personal autonomy to refuse medical treatment does not turn on wisdom, i.e., medical rationality...because health care decisions intrinsically concern one's subjective sense of well-being.... [T]he state has not embraced an unqualified or undifferentiated policy of preserving life at the expense of personal autonomy.... As a general proposition, the notion that the individual exists for the good of the state is, of course, quite antithetical to our fundamental thesis that the role of the state is to ensure a maximum of individual freedom of choice and conduct.[32]

The language of these decisions is clear. Yet, the decisions have made no dent in the fortress that is psychiatric slavery. On the contrary, they have been used, as I showed elsewhere, to reinforce that fortress by corrupting the principle of autonomy.[33] The result is that, since World War II, celebrated "psychiatric abuses"—exemplified by the "snake pits"—have seemingly disappeared from the American scene. Yet, during the same period, the power of psychiatry as a *de facto* arm of the coercive apparatus of the state underwent an explosive growth and has become a veritable Leviathan, the foundation and main executive arm of the Therapeutic State.

Conclusion

The difficulty with lofty moral principles is that it is easy to enunciate them but difficult to abide by them. Such is the case with the principles of nonaggression and self-ownership. Both are too demanding. They require us to respect others, and to expect others to respect us. They demand that we hold ourselves responsible for what we do, and hold others responsible for what they do. In short, they require us to treat people better than in fact they are. But would we consider a moral principle lofty if it did not require us to do just that? Only by treating men better than they are can they become better than they were. As Johann Wolfgang von Goethe (1749-1832) wisely observed: "If I accept you as you are, I will make you worse; however, if I treat you as though you are what you are capable of becoming, I help you become that."[34] Happily, man's reach for doing the right thing has always exceeded his grasp. Perhaps therein lies the engine of moral progress.

On the economic front, libertarians have fought a successful battle against centralized power and have secured a solid beachhead for the "free market." The most important challenge now facing libertarians lies, in my view, on the psychiatric front—that is, abolishing coercive or involuntary psychiatry root and branch and replacing it with a fully voluntary, contractual, "free market psychiatry," neither helped nor hindered by the state.

3

Economics and Psychiatry: Twin Scientisms

Prior to the Enlightenment, the marriage of church and state justified and implemented the coercive control of people by popes and princes. As the authority of the church declined, two new institutions—economics and psychiatry, each typically married to the state—assumed the role of justifying and legitimating social controls. One rationalizes abridging people's freedom by economic regulation, epitomized by taxation. The other justifies abridging people's freedom by psychiatric regulation, epitomized by the diagnosis and treatment of mental illness.

Scientists have long agreed that, qua scientists, they deal with *how things are*, not with how they ought to be. Science is peaceful. Its methods are careful observation, experimentation, reflection, study, verification, falsification. Fraud and force have no legitimate place in the practice of science. In contrast, religion and politics deal with how *people ought to live in society*, not with human anatomy or physiology. Fraud and force are integral to their practices.

The study of the consequences of economic policies and medical treatments belongs to science. The implementation of rules to promote certain behaviors and prohibit others belongs to religion and politics.

The success of science has inevitably spawned imitations of science, called "scientisms." The term is of recent origin. The *Oxford English Dictionary* dates its first appearance to 1877 and defines scientism thus: "The habit and mode of expression of a man of science." I regard scientism as a type of cheating or impersonation—a nonscientist pretending to be a scientist. This description fits both economists and psychiatrists perfectly.

In the natural sciences—astronomy, physics, and chemistry—regularities and relations between phenomena are formulated in mathematical or other specialized symbolic notation, rather than in ordinary language.[1]

Imitating real scientists, economists and psychiatrists use (pseudo) scientific language, but cannot dispense with the use of ordinary language as well. The scientific-scientistic language of economics is mathematics, of psychiatry, neuroscience. That is for show. The real action lies in law and politics: economists and psychiatrists solicit politicians to enact the kinds of economic and psychiatric policies they favor. In both cases, leaders devote their energies to seeking support from politicians, philanthropists, and industrialists, and let the less prominent members of the profession serve the needs of clients.

In this chapter, I show that the functions of both economics and psychiatry are, properly speaking, theological and political. Both deal with beliefs and values; both offer explanations of how people live and recommendations of how they ought to live; and both use force and justify its use by professional rhetoric.[2]

Economics as Rhetoric and Religion

Robert H. Nelson, professor of economics at the University of Maryland School of Public Affairs, titles his most recent book *Economics as Religion*.[3] He writes:

> Economists think of themselves as scientists, but as I will be arguing in this book, they are more like theologians.... [A] basic role of economists is to serve as the priesthood of a modern secular religion of economic progress that serves many of the same functions in contemporary society as earlier Christian and other religions did in their time.... Beneath the surface of their formal economic theorizing, economists are engaged in an act of delivering religious messages. Correctly understood, these messages are seen to be promises of the true path to a salvation in this world—to a new heaven on earth. Because this path follows along a route of economic progress, and because economists are the ones—or so it is believed by many people—with the technical understanding to show the way, it falls to the members of the economics profession (assisted by other social scientists) to assume the traditional role of the priesthood."[4]

This thesis complements my view of psychiatry as religion, rhetoric, and repression.[5] I maintain that the medical scaffolding that supports psychiatry as an institution of medical healing is a myth. Nelson maintains that the mathematical scaffolding that supports economics as a science is a myth:

> To be sure, economics may perform a valuable social role without adding any significant understanding to the knowledge of the economy—a "good myth," economically speaking, can work not only in primitive tribal cultures but also in modern societies. In this respect, Samuelson might be judged a large scientific failure and a great religious and economic success.... If we penetrate below the surface in this way, [Paul A. Samuelson's] *Economics* [1948] is revealed to be a religious work grounded in articles of progressive faith, as well as conventional economic forces at work.[6]

Ironically, it was John Maynard Keynes (1883-1946)—the most famous twentieth-century economist, harsh critic of Austrian economics, and himself a competent mathematician—who, as early as 1936, cautioned: "Too large a proportion of recent 'mathematical' economics are mere concoctions, as imprecise as the initial assumptions they rest on, which allow the author to lose sight of the complexities and interdependencies of the real world in a maze of pretentious and unhelpful symbols."[7]

Many mathematicians agree. Norbert Wiener (1894-1964)—professor of mathematics at the Massachusetts Institute of Technology (MIT) and a founder of cybernetics—offered this critique of the fakeries of mathematical economics:

> Mathematical physics has come to be one of the great triumphs of modern times.... The success of mathematical physics has led the social scientist to be jealous of its power without quite understanding the intellectual attitudes that had contributed to this power. The use of mathematical formulae had accompanied the development of the natural sciences and become the mode in the social sciences. *Just as primitive peoples adopt the Western modes of denationalized clothing and of parliamentarianism out of a vague feeling that these magic rites and vestments will at once put them abreast of modern culture and technique, so the economists have developed the habit of dressing up their rather imprecise ideas in the language of the infinitesimal calculus. In doing this, they show scarcely more discrimination than some of the emerging African nations in the assertion of their rights....* An econometrician will develop an elaborate and ingenious theory of demand and supply, inventories and unemployment, and the like, with a relative or total indifference to the methods by which these elusive quantities are observed or measured.... To assign what purports to be precise values to such essentially vague quantities is neither useful nor honest, and *any pretense of applying precise formulae to these loosely defined quantities is a sham and waste of time.*[8]

In his 1974 Nobel Banquet address, which I shall consider in the next chapter, Friedrich A. Hayek voiced the same criticism.[9] In 1993, libertarian economist and social critic Robert Higgs offered this reminiscence of his subjection to indoctrination into the arcana of Samuelson's economics:

> Like most graduate students in economics during the last 40 years, I spent many painful hours plowing through Paul Samuelson's *Foundations of Economic Analysis* (Harvard University Press, 1947). From that sacred text we novices learned how to prove many specific theorems. Far more important, *we learned how neoclassical economics—"modern economic science"—was supposed to be done.* We built mathematically specified "models," sets of equations describing the relations of selected economic variables.... Playing increasingly clever mathematical tricks with the models constituted "scientific progress."

Samuelson fashioned his models, which set the standard, after 19th-century physics.... Economics was reduced to various types of the same calculus problem: finding a constrained *extremum*. The economist's job was to state the objective function and the constraints, then grind out the solutions.... By the 1960s, if not earlier, academic economists who quarreled with this way of doing the job were...regarded by mainstream neoclassical economists as defenders of lost causes or as kooks, misguided critics, and antiscientific oddballs. By aping 19th-century physicists, neoclassical economists *convinced themselves and others that they were doing science, but the effort was basically misguided, not so much scientific as, in F. A. Hayek's term, "scientistic."*[10]

In 1976, writing about drug prohibition, I suggested that we distinguish between ceremonial and technical performances, roles, and functions: the function of the priestly garb is ceremonial; that of the surgical glove and gown, technical.[11] The German free-market economist Wilhelm Röpke (1899-1966) offered this witty account of "ceremonial economics":

It is a serious misunderstanding to wish to defend the mathematical method with the argument that economics has to do with quantities. That is true, but it is true also of strategy, and yet battles are not mathematical problems to be entrusted to an electronic computer. The crucial things in economics are about as mathematically intractable as a love letter or a Christmas celebration.... [O]nly too often does mathematical economics resemble the children's game of hiding Easter eggs, great jubilation breaking out when the eggs are found precisely where they were hidden—a witty simile which we owe to the contemporary economist L. Albert Hahn. The same irreverence, I am afraid, is due mathematical economics when it pretends to furnish us precise results.... We reply that it is better to be imprecisely right than to be precisely wrong.[12]

In this connection, D. N. McCloskey's work—especially *The Rhetoric of Economics* (1985)—deserves special mention.[13] In an essay entitled "The rhetoric of economic development," McCloskey observed: "It is not surprising that economics, taking itself to be social engineering, should lose its way. Economics around 1950 gave up social philosophy and social history to become a blackboard subject. In the name of 'Science,' that magic English word, the scope of economic conversation was narrowed.... [Governments] were dazzled by Scientism, a world religion for a time in the mid-20th century."[14] Governments, and not only governments, are still dazzled by it and are likely to be dazzled for as long as science remains such a useful tool for improving the material conditions of life.

McCloskey identifies economics as a type of "social self-understanding (a critical theory, indeed, like Marxism or psychoanalysis)" and mocks its "positivist ceremonial.... Most journals of economics nowadays look like journals of applied mathematics or theoretical statistics."[15] Peter Bauer and Wilhelm Röpke made virtually identical comments.

> Bauer: Mathematization of the subject has perhaps been the most conspicuous thread running through economics since I first encountered it. In the 1930s one could read the journals without much knowledge of mathematics.... Today one is regarded as unqualified without some knowledge of mathematics, and especially of its language.... Reading the journals one gets the impression that economics has become little more than a branch of applied mathematics and one that can be successfully pursued with little reference to real life phenomena.[16]

> Röpke: When one tries to read an economic journal nowadays, often enough one wonders whether one has not inadvertently picked up a journal of chemistry or hydraulics.... Economics is no natural science; it is a moral science and as such has to do with man as a spiritual and moral being.[17]

Most journals of psychiatry nowadays look like journals of neuroanatomy and pharmacology. And psychiatry is neither medicine nor a science.

Economists and psychiatrists both claim that they can make "scientifically reliable" predictions, the former about economic trends or markets, the latter about the dangerousness of psychiatric patients and the safety of psychiatric drugs. McCloskey disagrees: "Prediction is not possible in economics.... [P]redicting the economic future is, as Ludwig von Mises put it, 'beyond the power of any mortal man.'"[18] With cool irony, he notes that if economists knew the future, they could quickly accumulate "the unlimited wealth that such a Faustian knowledge [could] bring. He [the economist] is willing for some reason instead to dissipate the opportunity by the act of telling others about it."[19]

His following lines summarize the rhetorical similarities between economics and psychiatry: "Linguistics is an appropriate model for economic science.... It is perhaps clear by now that economists use rhetorical means to achieve their ends.... The persuasive cure [of economic scientism] is literary and rhetorical."[20]

A few more words regarding the similarities between economics and psychiatry and their respective pretenses to science are in order here. Although Ludwig von Mises was blind to the nature of the psychiatric enterprise, he pinpointed the complementary character of the two professions when he wrote: "Economics is not about things and tangible material objects; it is about men, their meanings and actions.... The notions of abnormality and perversity therefore have no place in economics."[21]

Mises seems to be assigning the job of identifying and describing human behavior to economics, and the job of evaluating and classifying it as normal and abnormal to psychiatry. Actually, both disciplines do both things.

Friedrich von Wieser (1851-1926)—Mises's mentor and one of the founders of Austrian economics—also viewed economics as similar to psychology (psychiatry). He stated: "This investigation uses the methods recently designated as 'psychological.' The name is applied because the theory takes its point of departure from within, from the mind of economic man. I myself once spoke of economic theory in this sense as applied psychology."[22]

In a similar vein, Frank H. Knight (1885-1972), a cofounder (with Jacob Viner) of the "Chicago School" of economics, wrote: "Economics describes 'economic' behavior and an 'economic' social organization, insofar as human conduct conforms to certain rules, assumed to be known axiomatically, but not excluding other motives. Since its root idea is 'economy,' which is relative to *intentions* and these are not observed by the senses, it is *not* a strictly empirical or inductive science."[23] Psychiatrists are also in the business of studying and claiming to be experts on intentions and motives, *especially of other persons whom they call "mentally ill."*

The political character of economics is officially recognized and is reflected in the term "political economy." Free market economists are especially candid about this. Psychiatrists consider acknowledging the political character of their interventions taboo. They call depriving people of liberty "hospitalization" and insist that coercion is "treatment." To call psychiatry "political" is an insult to psychiatrist. They maintain it is "medical."

Still, the differences between economics and psychiatry as ostensibly and overtly scientific pursuits, but actually and covertly policy-making and policy-enforcing enterprises, remain and are reflected in the kinds of work for which investigators are awarded Nobel Prizes for contributions in these fields.

Nobel Prizes in "Economic Sciences"

The first Nobel Prizes were awarded in 1901. From then until 1969, the Prizes were given for achievements in physics, chemistry, medicine, literature, and peace. In 1968, the Bank of Sweden established "the Prize in Economic Sciences in memory of Alfred Nobel, founder of the Nobel Prize," generally called the "Nobel Prize in Economics."

The Prizes in Literature and Peace, not given for scientific work, do not concern us here. Neither do the Prizes in Physics and Chemistry, because these endeavors exemplify science. I am interested here in the Prizes in economics and in psychiatry-as-medicine. How is the awarding of these Prizes rationalized? The Prize in economics is rationalized by the mathematical and probabilistic apparatus that ostensibly undergirds the economist's work. *Mutatis mutandis*, the Prize in medicine/psychiatry is rationalized by the references to neuroanatomy, neurophysiology, neuropharmacology, and genetics that ostensibly form the scientific bases of the psychiatrist's therapeutic endeavors. In other words, mathematics is used to conceal the political nature of "economic science," neuromythology and pharmacomythology to conceal the political nature of "psychiatric science."

The first Nobel Prize in Economics, in 1969, was awarded to Ragnar Frisch and Jan Tirbergen, for "having developed and applied dynamic models for the analysis of economic processes." In 1970, the recipient was Paul A. Samuelson, honored "for the scientific work through which he has developed static and dynamic economic theory and actively contributed to raising the level of analysis in economic science."[24] The 1971 winner, Simon Kuznets, was honored for his "empirically founded interpretation of economic growth." The winners in 1972, Sir John R. Hicks and Kenneth J. Arrow, received the Prize for their "pioneering contributions to general economic equilibrium theory and welfare theory." In 1973, Wassily Leontieff was honored for "developing the input-output method and for its application to important economic problems." Every one of these men was a practitioner of mathematical economics and, not coincidentally, an advocate of socialist, command-control economies.

In 1974, the Prize was divided between Gunnar Myrdal and Friedrich A. von Hayek, for their "pioneering work in the theory of money and economic fluctuations and for their penetrating analysis of the interdependence of economic, social and institutional phenomena."[25] Karl Gunnar Myrdal (1898-1987)—an outspoken socialist prominent in Swedish politics—had served as executive secretary of the United Nations Economics Commission for Europe. Hayek—the first free market economist to receive the Prize—stood for everything Myrdal opposed. I discuss Hayek's views in a separate chapter.[26] Two years later, when Milton Friedman received the Prize, Gunnar Myrdal declared that "the economics prize should be removed because it had been given to such reactionaries as Friedman and Hayek."[27]

Some of the other winners of the economics Prize and their work deserve to be briefly mentioned. In 1990, the Prize was awarded to three Americans, Harry M. Markowitz, Merton H. Miller, and William F. Sharpe, for their work in "the theory of financial economics," that is, the economics of investing, by both individuals and institutions. The names of all three men, especially Markowitz's, are associated with what has become known as "Modern Portfolio Theory." Characterized as "the philosophical opposite of traditional stock picking," in Modern Portfolio Theory, "investments are described statistically, in terms of their expected long-term return rate and their expected short-term volatility.... The goal is to identify your acceptable level of risk tolerance, and then to find a portfolio with the maximum expected return for that level of risk."[28]

Identifying a person's "acceptable level of risk tolerance" sounds like identifying his blood pressure. Of course, it is nothing of the sort. Making investing in commodities or stocks appear "scientific"—supposedly turning it into a "method" of successful investing—is like inventing the perpetual motion machine. It is, as Austrian economists have always maintained, a self-contradiction.[29] Simple observation of everyday life confutes the proposition. In physics, the individuals most successful at making, say, nuclear bombs or computers are scientists, not amateurs. In investing, speculators, such as a George Soros, are more successful than are professional economists.

The 1994 Nobel Prize in Economics was awarded to three men for mathematical work in economics. They were John C. Harsanyi, Reinhard Selten, and John F. Nash, Jr. Harsanyi was a mathematical economist, Selten and Nash were mathematicians. Nash's story is of special interest. The combination of Nash's psychiatric history with his receiving the Nobel Prize led writer Sylvia Nasar to compose an excellent biography of him, making Nash one of the best known Nobel Laureates in the world—not for his work, but for his being "a schizophrenic."[30] In his acceptance speech for the Prize, Nash stated:

> Now I must arrive at the time of my change from scientific rationality of thinking into the delusional thinking characteristic of persons who are psychiatrically diagnosed as "schizophrenic" or "paranoid schizophrenic." But I will not really attempt to describe this long period of time but rather avoid *embarrassment* by simply omitting to give the details of truly personal type.... The mental disturbances originated in the early months of 1959 at a time when *Alicia [Nash's wife] happened to be pregnant*. And as a consequence I resigned my position as a faculty member at M.I.T. and, ultimately, after spending 50 days under "observation" at the McLean Hospital, traveled to Europe and attempted to gain status there as a refugee. I later spent times of

the order of five to eight months in hospitals in New Jersey, *always on an involuntary basis and always attempting a legal argument for release.* And it did happen that when I had been long enough hospitalized that I would finally *renounce* my delusional hypotheses and revert to thinking of myself as a human of more conventional circumstances and return to mathematical research.... Then gradually I began to intellectually reject some of the delusionally influenced lines of thinking which had been characteristic of my orientation.... So at the present time I seem to be thinking rationally again in the style that is characteristic of scientists. *However this is not entirely a matter of joy as if someone returned from physical disability to good physical health. One aspect of this is that rationality of thought imposes a limit on a person's concept of his relation to the cosmos.* For example, a non-Zoroastrian could think of Zarathustra as simply a madman who led millions of naive followers to adopt a cult of ritual fire worship. But without his "madness" Zarathustra would necessarily have been only another of the millions or billions of human individuals who have lived and then been forgotten.... [31]

This is not the place for me to comment on Nash's "illness" and "recovery," or his relationship to his wife and psychiatry. Suffice it to note that, although the Nobel Committee, the American Psychiatric Association, Nash, Nasar, and every major social institution in Western society maintains that schizophrenia is a bona fide brain disease, Nash refers to its details as "embarrassments." Also, a careful reader of Nasar's biography might reasonably conclude that Nash did not *happen* to reject his role obligations as husband and impending father "precisely at the time when Alicia happened to be pregnant," as he puts it. He did not simply "break down." He "fled" to Europe. Alicia went after him, with great effort found him, brought him back, repeatedly committed him, and gave consent to his being "treated" with both insulin shock and electroshock. Nash speaks bitterly about his commitments and "treatments."

The 2002 Economics Prize was shared by Daniel Kahneman and Vernon L. Smith. Kahneman, a psychologist, was cited for his contributions to economic science based on "insight from psychology": "Traditionally, much of economic research has relied on the assumption of a '*homo œconomicus*' motivated by self-interest and capable of rational decision-making.... Daniel Kahneman has integrated insights from psychology into economics, thereby laying the foundation for a new field of research. Kahneman's main findings concern decision-making under uncertainty, where he has demonstrated how human decisions may systematically depart from those predicted by standard economic theory."[32]

Daniel Altman, the business reporter for the *New York Times*, explained Kahneman's discoveries as follows:

> Professor Kahneman made the economically puzzling discovery that most of his subjects would make a 20-minute trip to buy a calculator for $10 instead of $15, but would not make the same trip to buy a jacket for $120 instead of $125—saving the same $5.... "Kahneman's a psychologist—he's interested in *how your brain works*, how you make decisions," said Alvin E. Roth, an economist at Harvard who specializes in experimental methods.[33]

Note that a professor of economics at Harvard, Alvin E. Roth, believes that a psychologist who asks students about how much travel time they would be willing to sacrifice to save a small sum is using a *scientific method for studying how the brain works.*

In the *Daily Princetonian*, Joshua Tauberer, the interviewer, explained Kahneman's prizewinning work as,

> an attempt to provide a more realistic set of ideas for what the economic agent is really like.... In one of Kahneman's studies, he gave half of the participants a mug and the other half no mug. The results showed that people with a mug wanted to trade the mug for an average of approximately $7 cash, while the people without a mug valued the same type of mug at $3 cash. The two acts are logically the same—trading a mug for money—Kahneman explained, but those with mugs did not want to give up something they already had. This "very myopic" aspect of human decision making was, when Kahneman first started this line of research in 1969, not a widely accepted part of economic theory. One of Kahneman's initial papers on this subject...was published in an economics journal rather than a psychology journal. *Though that decision was "quite accidental," it might have been the reason he was accepting the Nobel Prize yesterday, Kahneman said.*[34]

Kahneman's "research" is both trivial and mischievous: trivial, because we have long known that a bird in the hand is worth two in the bush; mischievous, because it promotes the view that people are "irrational." Common belief in miracles, supernatural phenomena, and revealed religion in general ought to be evidence enough that the terms "rational" and "irrational" lack the kind of precision we associate with scientific discourse.

Closely related to the Kahneman-type psychological economics is so-called "behavioral finance," which "teaches that stock market investors are irrational."[35] Writers who use the terms "rational/irrational" do not bother to define them; instead, they illustrate them, typically with examples that are existentially "rational," albeit economically "irrational."

Richard Thaler, characterized by *Fortune* as a pioneer in "behavioral economics," asked a few friends "how much they'd be willing to pay to eliminate a one-in-1,000 chance of immediate death and how much they would have to be paid to willingly accept an extra one-in-1,000 chance of immediate death. What he found was that they wouldn't pay much for the extra margin of safety but demanded huge sums to accept added risk—which isn't, strictly speaking, rational."[36] Thaler's question poses an existential, not a logical, problem. Calling the behavior "irrational" interferes with our understanding of it, the same way as, for example, calling a mother who kills her children "insane" interferes with our understanding of her behavior.

The reporter for *Fortune* quotes Thaler stating, "The disparity between buying and selling prices was very interesting," and adds, "Thaler did discuss his subversive thoughts with a few trusted colleagues."[37] This is a *subversive thought*? The *Fortune* article's conclusion resonates revealingly with the psychiatrist's mandate to protect the patient from himself: "[M]uch of what the behavioralists [sic] have to offer in terms of advice has to do with *protecting retail investors from themselves.*"[38]

Humorists have long seen through the phoniness of this kind of "research," for which it is not really necessary to perform experiments. An old Jewish joke, which I cite from memory, is an example:

> At the beginning of a first-grade class, the teacher wants to determine what the children in her class know and don't know. She asks if anyone knows how to add. Many hands go up. Then she asks if anyone knows how to multiply. Only one hand goes up, little Sammy Cohen's. The teacher asks: "Sammy, can you tell me how much is 3 times 4?" Sammy replies: "Well, that depends. Are you buying or selling?"

The proposition that people are irrational is an idea that has long been dear to the hearts of psychiatrists and psychoanalysts. The very title of Freud's famous book, *The Psychopathology of Everyday Life*, entails this view.[39]

Nobel Prizes in "Psychiatric Sciences"

Only five researchers have received the Nobel Prize for contributions to the medical specialty called "psychiatry," and only one was a psychiatrist or, more precisely, a neuropsychiatrist. Julius Wagner-Jauregg (1857-1940), a professor of psychiatry at the University of Vienna, was honored in 1927 "for his discovery of the therapeutic value of malaria inoculation in the treatment of dementia paralytica." Dementia paralytica, also known as general paralysis of the insane or paresis, is a late manifestation of syphilis. Wagner-Jauregg's discovery was a contribution to the treatment of an infectious illness, not a "mental" illness. The treatment was rendered obsolete by the discovery of antibiotics. The discovery had no political or civil rights implications.

In 1949, the Portuguese neurologist and neurosurgeon Antonio Caetano de Abreu Freire Egas Moniz (1874-1955) was awarded the Nobel Prize in Medicine for the invention of lobotomy as an effective treatment for psychoses. The term "psychosis" does not name an objectively identifiable disease. Moniz's patients were persons incarcerated in mental hospitals, treated against their will. In his presentation speech, Herbert Olivecrona, a professor at the Royal Caroline Institute and the most famous neurosurgeon of his day, lauded Moniz with these words:

> The lines of thought along which Antonio Egas Moniz has advanced to the discovery of the prefrontal leucotomy refer primarily to the localization of certain psychic functions in the brain. It has long been known that the frontal lobes are of great importance for higher cerebral activity, especially in regard to the emotions.... It occurred to Moniz that *psychic morbid states* accompanied by affective tension might be relieved by *destroying* the frontal lobes or their connections to other parts of the brain. On the basis of this idea Moniz gradually worked out an operative method whose purpose was to interrupt the lines of communication of the frontal lobes to the rest of the brain.... It was soon found that morbid conditions in which emotional tension was a dominating part of the pathological picture reacted very favorably to such operations. *To this group of diseases belong, primarily, states of depression accompanied by fear and anxiety, obsessive neuroses, certain forms of persecution mania, and a considerable part of the most important and common of all mental diseases, schizophrenia: those cases, namely, in which the schizophrenic pattern of behaviour and the emotional condition is affectively charged to a high degree, as for instance in states of anguish or anxiety, refusal to take food, aggressiveness, and the like.* Great subjective suffering and invalidism are characteristic of this group of diseases. *Many of the diseased, especially within the schizophrenic group, are very difficult patients and are often dangerous to the people around them....*[40]

Three of the most famous American victims of this atrocity are Rosemary Kennedy, sister of President John F. Kennedy and Senator Edward Kennedy; Rose Williams, the sister of Tennessee Williams; and film star Frances Farmer.[41]

In 1949, when the Nobel committee awarded the Prize to Moniz, it took for granted that the phenomena psychiatrists call "schizophrenia" are the manifestations of a brain disease. Fifty years later, the committee takes for granted that all (major) mental illnesses are diseases of the brain, in the same sense as, say, Parkinsonism is a disease of the brain. These assumptions may turn out to be the greatest and most characteristic delusions of our age.[42]

The 2000 Prize in Medicine was shared by three men—Arvid Carlsson, Paul Greengard, and Eric R. Kandel—"for their discoveries concerning signal transduction in the nervous system" and for "an understanding of the normal function of the brain and how disturbances in this signal transduction can give rise to neurological and *psychiatric diseases. These findings have resulted in the development of new drugs.*"[43] The citation for Carlsson, a Swedish physician-pharmacologist, stated:

> Arvid Carlsson, Department of Pharmacology, Göteborg University is rewarded for his discovery that dopamine is a transmitter in the brain and that it has great importance for our ability to control movements. His research has led to the realization that Parkinson's disease is caused by a lack of dopamine in certain parts of the brain and that an efficient remedy (L-dopa) for this disease could be developed.... He showed that antipsychotic drugs, mostly used against schizophrenia, affect synaptic transmission by blocking dopamine receptors. The discoveries of Arvid Carlsson have had great importance for *the treatment of depression, which is one of our most common diseases.* He has contributed strongly to the development of selective serotonin uptake blockers, a new generation of antidepressive drugs.[44]

The Nobel committee legitimized depression as a disease on a par with diabetes and placed its stamp of approval on the use of antidepressants as a form of medical treatment on a par with the use of antibiotics. Parkinsonism is a proven brain disease, treated by neurologists. To my knowledge, no patient with Parkinsonism is forced to take an anti-Parkinson drug against his will. Depression and schizophrenia are mental diseases, not proven brain diseases, treated by psychiatrists. Patients with such diagnoses are regularly forced to take antipsychotic drugs, a fact that is evidently of no concern to the savants at the Karolinska Institute.

From a psychiatric point of view, the most interesting figure among the three winners of the 2000 Prize in Medicine is Eric R. Kandel. Born in Vienna, Kandel and his family emigrated to the United States just before the outbreak of World War II. Kandel received a medical degree and, intending to become a psychoanalyst, was trained in psychiatry. He then switched fields and devoted his career to basic research in the biology of the nervous system, mainly in the simple organism, the sea slug. In his autobiography, prepared for the Nobel committee, Kandel wrote:

> I entered N.Y.U. Medical School dedicated to studying psychiatry and becoming a psychoanalyst. Although I stayed with this career plan through my

internship and psychiatric residency, by my senior year in medical school I had become so interested in the biological basis of medical practice (as had everyone else in my class) that I decided I had to learn something about the biology of the mind.... [S]everal psychoanalysts...had begun to discuss the potential importance of the biology of the brain for the future of psycho-analysis.[45]

The Nobel committee summarized the work for which Kandel was honored as follows:

Eric Kandel, Center for Neurobiology and Behavior, Columbia University, New York, is rewarded for his discoveries of how the efficiency of synapses can be modified, and which molecular mechanisms that take part.... The fundamental mechanisms that Eric Kandel has revealed [in the sea slug] are also applicable to humans.... Even if the road towards an understanding of complex memory functions still is long, the results of Eric Kandel have provided a critical building stone. It is now possible to continue and for instance study how complex memory images are stored in our nervous system, and how it is possible to recreate the memory of earlier events....[46]

Kandel is a true believer in biological psychiatry and a faithful practitioner of the politically correct silence concerning the human rights violations endemic to its practice. In an article entitled "A new intellectual framework for psychiatry," published in the *American Journal of Psychiatry* in 1998, he explained:

This framework can be summarized in five principles.... Principle 1. *All mental processes, even the most complex psychological processes, derive from operations of the brain. The central tenet of this view is that what we commonly call mind is a range of functions carried out by the brain.... As a corollary, behavioral disorders that characterize psychiatric illness are disturbances of brain function, even in those cases where the causes of the disturbances are clearly environmental in origin....* Principle 5. *Insofar as psychotherapy or counseling is effective and produces long-term changes in behavior, it presumably does so through learning, by producing changes in gene expression that alter the strength of synaptic connections and structural changes that alter the anatomical pattern of interconnections between nerve cells of the brain....* All Functions of Mind Reflect Functions of Brain.... As is now evident in DSM-IV, the classification of mental disorders must be based on criteria other than the presence or absence of gross anatomical abnormalities. *The absence of detectable structural changes does not rule out the possibility that more subtle but nonetheless important biological changes are occurring.*[47]

None of this is new, or true. Theodor Meynert (1833-1892), one of the founders of modern neuropsychiatry, began his textbook, *Psychiatry*

(1884), with this statement: "The reader will find no other definition of 'Psychiatry' in this book but the one given on the title page: *Clinical Treatise on Diseases of the Forebrain.* The historical term for psychiatry, i.e., 'treatment of the soul,' implies more than we can accomplish, and transcends the bounds of accurate scientific investigation."[48]

Kandel lets neither political nor psychiatric history interfere with his enthusiasm for preaching the gospel that the brain secretes thought like the kidney secretes urine. In an interview, he explained:

> "I went into the biology of memory because I was looking for a problem that was at once deep and yet amenable to a reductionist approach relevant to psychiatry," he says. Healthy behavioral changes rely on memory and learning.... Kandel pointed out in his 1998 article that Freud himself originally sought "a neural model of behavior in an attempt to develop a scientific psychology."... *The advent of effective psychiatric drugs in the last three decades forced psychiatry to confront neuroscience.... Imaging technology, for example, has the potential to do away with the differentiation between "organic" conditions, marked by obvious brain lesions, and "functional" ones, which so far are reflected solely in behavior.* "Insofar as psychotherapy works," Kandel explains, it's got to be doing something [in the brain].... So then the question is what is most effective for a particular patient," Kandel says. Cognitive neuroscience and molecular biology thus may be able to identify the physical structures and biochemical signaling systems of the brain that are associated with the various components of the classical psychoanalytical model of the mind.... [T]o those who fear he is reducing the psychiatric patient to a set of biological functions, Kandel replies, "The patient is a set of biological functions," and then laughs again.[49]

Kandel calls "psychiatric drugs" "effective," as if that were a fact. Actually, only some psychiatric drugs are effective, and they are effective only in making the patient's behavior more acceptable to his family or psychiatrist. No psychiatric drug can be said to be truly effective as long as we lack objective markers for the diseases they allegedly treat. Kandel also proclaims his version of a simplistic biological reductionism and gratuitously pontificates about the evils of private profit: "Like all knowledge, biological knowledge is a double-edged sword. It can be used for ill as well as for good, *for private profit or public benefit....* Brain sciences have also been and can again be misused for social control and manipulation.... The only way to encourage the responsible use of this knowledge is *to base the uses of biology in social policy on an understanding of biology.*"[50]

It is saddening to hear such words from a person who was himself a refugee from a "social policy [based] on an understanding of biology."

We also learn that, notwithstanding Kandel's condemnation of "private profit," he and his colleagues are turning their work into just that: "Three men who shared the 2000 Nobel Prize for unraveling the mysteries of the brain...[have become] entrepreneurs, each starting a biotechnology company."[51]

Neuroeconomics: Bewitchment with Neuroscientism

It is naive to believe that the fashionable scientific model of a particular age—cosmological, horological, electronic, or neurobiological—can explain human action. It cannot. The modern neuroscientistic search for the seat of the mind as choice-maker is but a new version of the medieval scholar's search for the seat of the soul performing that function. Descartes located the soul in the pineal gland. When science displaced religion, the mind replaced the soul and people began to look for the seat of the mind. Not surprisingly, they found it in the brain, rediscovering the "discovery" of the great pagan physician, Hippocrates, who stated: "Men ought to know that from nothing else but the brain come joy, despondency and lamentation.... By the same organ we become mad and delirious, and fears and terrors assail us."[52]

I am not the first, and will not be the last, to lament the modern mind's bewitchment with scientism, whose promises and perils are equally obvious. Mathematics, the language of the natural sciences, is indeed a useful tool: it enables us to see what is otherwise invisible. Metaphors, the language of the social sciences, may easily do the opposite. Confused with things, metaphors may prevent us from seeing the obvious. This is why in the natural sciences knowledge can be gained only with the mastery of their special languages. Whereas in human affairs, knowledge can be gained only by mastering the subtleties of ordinary language and seeing through the rhetoric of religion, politics, and psychiatry.

Because the measurement of quantities expressible in mathematical terms has served as the basis of the natural sciences, the scientism of the social sciences was first based on imitating mathematics by adopting the use of its methods. Psychiatrists and psychologists created psychometrics, the psychological theory and technique of mental measurement, and economists created econometrics, the application of statistical methods to the study of economic data and problems.

Modern psychiatric scientism is based on neurologizing behavior. As this trend gained momentum, the prefix "neuro-" became endowed with magical rhetorical powers. To make an activity or intervention sci-entific—and to lend support to the claim that mental illnesses are brain diseases—it is enough to give it a name that begins with this fashionable prefix. In addition to neuroanatomy, neurophysiology, and neurosurgery, we now speak of neuroleptic drugs, neuroradiological studies, neuropsy-chological tests, neurotransmitters, neurochemicals, neuropharmacology, neurobiology, neuroscience, neurolinguistics, neuroethics, neurophilos-ophy, neuro-epistemology, and—behold—neuroeconomics.

What is neuroeconomics? It is a farcical effort to gain scientific legiti-macy for economics by reducing commercial behavior to neuroanatomy and neurophysiology. According to Paul Zak, professor of economics at Claremont Graduate University in Claremont, California, "Just as mainstream psychology started looking for brain-based explanations of behavior, so is mainstream economics.... To understand economic deci-sions, you need to understand the brain.... One promise of neuroeconomics is revealing the basis for 'irrational' financial behavior."[53] The assertion, "To understand economic decisions, you need to understand the brain...," is nonsense. If it were true, we would need to "understand the brain" in order to understand not only economic decisions, but also moral, political, mathematical, personal, and every other kind of decisions.

As I see it, neuroeconomics is a pseudoscience, ostensibly based on neuroradiology, proving that economic choices are illusions. We don't make choices, our brains do. The reports of science writers about this business are astonishingly uncritical. Sandra Blakeslee, who writes for the *New York Times*, explains:

> [R]esearchers are busy scanning the brains of people as they make economic decisions, barter, compete, cooperate, defect, punish, engage in auctions, gam-ble and calculate their next economic moves. *Based on their understanding of how fluctuations in neurons and brain chemicals drive those behaviors, the neuroscientists are expressing their findings in differential equations and other mathematical language beloved by economists....* The brain needs a way to compare and evaluate objects, people, events, memories, internal states and the perceived needs of others so that *it can make choices.* It does so by assigning relative value to everything that happens. But instead of dollars and cents, the brain relies on the firing rates of a number of *neurotransmitters—the chem-icals, like dopamine, that transmit nerve impulses....* Bullish investors have different patterns of dopamine release compared with bearish investors....[54]

Since there are no tests for measuring "patterns of dopamine release," researchers cannot know this, and it is the duty of science writers to point this out.

Sharon Begley's account, in the *Wall Street Journal Europe*, is similarly sensationalistic. She writes: "At a brain-imaging center in Massachusetts, a team of scientists that includes one of this year's Nobel laureates in economics, makes functioning resonance imaging [fMRI] scans of volunteers' brains. When people anticipate monetary rewards, the fMRI shows, the circuits that switch on are the very ones that go wild when you anticipate a delectable chocolate truffle, sex, or, in the case of addicts, cocaine.... *Welcome to neuroeconomics...[the] marriage of brain science and economics....* This year's economic Nobelists *recognized that economic decisions, like all others, reflect brain activity.*"[55]

Do all economists now *recognize* "that economic decisions, like all others, reflect brain activity"? If they do, they believe in a meaningless statement: If all decisions reflect brain activity, the assertion is as empty as asserting that everything we do depends on our having a body. If brain activity reveals the basis for *irrational* financial behavior, it must also reveal the basis for *rational* financial behavior: "fMRI scans show that trust is marked by high activity in two brain regions...." Do fMRI scans reveal trust in God as well as in economic rationality? Virginia Postrel, former editor of *Reason* magazine, enthuses:

> Why do people react differently to the same situation? And why do so many people give up money to punish anonymous cheapskates?... *Now a new field, called neuroeconomics, is using the tools of neuroscience to find the underlying biological mechanisms that lead people to act, or not act,* according to economic theory. In neuroeconomics, volunteers go through exercises developed by experimental economists studying trust or risk. Instead of simply observing subjects' behavior, however, *researchers use imaging technologies, like M.R.I.'s, to see which brain areas are active during the experiment.* "[Researchers] can predict with good reliability, from looking at the brain, what a person will do," said Colin F. Camerer, an economist at the California Institute of Technology....[56]

The claim that neuroscientists "can predict with good reliability, from looking at the brain, what a person will do," is a new version and reinforcement of the claim that psychiatrists can predict with good reliability, from looking at one or another "psychological test" or their "clinical examination," what a person will do. This piece of braggadocio would be laughable if it did not have the terrifying legal and social consequences it has.

Neuroeconomics *locates human action* in the brain much the same way that neurolinguistics *locates language in the brain*. The only question that remains is: Where? "Where in your brain is a word that you've learned?" asks the neurolinguist. "[I]f you know two languages, are they stored in two different parts of your brain?"[57] Neurolinguists claim expertise in special "methods" they call "neurolinguistic programming" and "neurolin-guistic deprogramm-ing," certify practitioners in these techniques, and make common professional cause with psychologists and hypnotists.

Conclusion

Mainstream (neoclassical) economists base their claim that economics is a science on mathematics: they use mathematical notation, equations and statistics, and formulate "economic laws." How can we reconcile mathematical "methodology" with the objects economists study, men in action? What part of mathematical economics is *functional*, relevant to what economists actually do, and what part is *ceremonial*, a means to lend their practices an aura of scientific respectability?[58] Since economists do many things, there is no single answer. However, many of the best known economists—for example, John Maynard Keynes, John Kenneth Galbraith, Milton Friedman—have become famous for their political, not their professional, contributions to the field.

Psychiatrists base their claim that psychiatry is a science on neuropathology, neuroscience, and psychopharmacology: they study the structure and function of the brain, treat (mis)behaviors as if they were brain diseases, and prescribe drugs for persons they diagnose as mentally ill. How can we reconcile the psychiatrists' professing neuroscience but practicing incarceration, forced drugging, and excuse-making?[59] What part of neuroscientific psychiatry is *functional*, relevant to what psychiatrists do, and what part is *ceremonial*, that is, a means to lend their practices an aura of scientific respectability? Everyone is free to answer this question for himself.

Why are economists and psychiatrists so eager to claim special scientific status for themselves? For the same reason that, formerly, priests claimed special theological status for themselves. Because they want to be able to sell their supposedly useful services to the public and the government; and, most importantly, by serving the state, they want to be in a position to influence its policies.

In theological-charitable states, clergymen justify the rule of the rulers. In therapeutic-welfare states, psychiatrists and economists perform the same function. Formerly, people believed that priests had special insights into the workings of heaven and earth. They didn't. Today, people believe that psychiatrists and neuroscientists have special insights into the "human mind." They don't.

4

Economocracy and Pharmacracy: Twin Systems of Social Control

In the previous chapter, I showed that economists and psychiatrists function as secular priests, social engineers, and agents of behavior control, but masquerade as scientists. In this chapter, I show that, perforce, economists and psychiatrists promote either coercion or cooperation—the individualist-capitalist market economy or the collectivist-therapeutic welfare economy; contractual-voluntary psychiatry or coercive-involuntary psychiatry. I illustrate and support this observation by describing the parallels between foreign aid and psychiatric aid (psychiatric services).

The Individual, the Family, and the State

Cooperation among persons and groups requires control of man's predatory impulses. Thus did the family, religion, and the state come into being, each assuming the task of controlling personal conduct.

As social beings, we must coordinate our behavior with the behavior of others, and vice versa. Such coordination is ensured by two means, external control or coercion and self-control or self-discipline. Persuasion and other forms of noncoercive influence are effective provided they succeed in altering the subject's choices. Some moral codes and political-economic systems value coercion by, and submission to, benevolent authorities more highly than they value self-control and independence, for example, theocracy, totalitarianism, and the therapeutic state. Others rank internal controls and voluntary cooperation more highly than external coercions, for example, the Protestant ethic, the market economy, and libertarianism.

Adam Smith—who taught moral philosophy, not economics—is revered as the prophet of the self-disciplined, cooperative lifestyle. For associations among adults, Smith advocated voluntary relations exemplified by trade, believing that, "When two men trade between themselves it is undoubtedly for the advantage of both."[1] Since the person "who is not disposed to respect the law and obey the civil magistrate" does not deserve the privileges of citizenship, Smith based his faith in cooperation on the premise that society will insure that, for the most part, its members are self-disciplined individuals.[2] In the Introduction I cited Burke's classic caveat, "Society cannot exist unless a controlling power upon will and appetite be placed somewhere, and the less there is within, the more there must be without. It is ordained in the eternal constitution of things, that men of intemperate minds cannot be free. Their passions forge their fetters."[3] I consider this observation so accurate and important that I believe we ought to call it the First Law of Political Philosophy.

From classical liberals like Adam Smith to modern libertarians like Ludwig von Mises, political philosophers recognized that human relations based on cooperation and contract—unlike those based on domination and coercion—presuppose and are contingent on the existence of independent, self-regulating actors. The libertarian prohibition against initiating the use of force does not apply to relations between certain caretakers and the persons who depend on them, especially infants, young children, and severely disabled persons. I begin by considering the situation of the child vis-à-vis his family and society and then examine the problem of disability.

In *Ecclesiastes* (3: 1-2), we read: "To every thing there is a season, and a time to every purpose under the heaven. A time to be born, and a time to die." For everyone, there is a time to be a child and depend on parents, a time to be an adult and be our parents' equal, and a time when we care for our parents as they had cared for us.

I use the words "child" and "childhood" to identify a biological condition of immaturity, a chronological condition of minority, and a socio-legal status of dependence on adults. Adults are larger, stronger, and more experienced than children, and can survive without them. Children cannot survive without adults. This basic inequality defines and shapes the child's relationship to the adult world.

In the modern West, childhood is, *inter alia*, a socio-legal status. The age at which that status ends and the status of adulthood begins varies depending on the context in which the issue of the person's minority status arises: it may be as low as ten or twelve, for being tried for a felony as an adult; fourteen or sixteen, for obtaining a limited driver's license; sixteen, for having the capacity to consent to sexual relations with an adult; eighteen, for voting and joining the military; twenty-one, for permission to purchase alcohol; and thirty-five, for eligibility for the presidency of the United States.

In the past, childhood ended much earlier than now with respect to certain activities, such as entering the labor force and marrying; while with respect to certain other activities, such as the right to own property or vote, it ended much later, or never.

To enable us to respect and obey ourselves, we must first learn to respect and obey our parents and parent surrogates. Because the family has proved to be the most effective social arrangement for transforming irresponsible children into responsible adults, it is our most enduring and most important social institution. For the same reason, hostility to the family has been the hallmark of the rhetoricians of political and therapeutic paternalism and totalitarianisms—Jacobins, Communists, Fascists, National Socialists, psychiatrists, social workers, and feminists. Each of these zealots and his cause masquerades as a "liberator" and form of "liberationism"; each seeks to destroy the family by blaming it for "causing" all manner of personal and social problems; and each seeks to replace the family by an authority whose legitimacy is based not on kinship but on "compassion," "science," or "therapy."

Adam Smith, too, was concerned about undermining the integrity of the family, albeit from a very different threat, namely, an excess of offspring. He warned that "where there are many children, they cannot all have the affection of the parent, and it is only by this means that any of them can establish themselves."[4]

Such considerations are a reminder of something obvious that, nevertheless, needs to be emphasized. I refer to the fact that libertarian principles are *principles*. They are not, and ought not to be confused with, a general philosophy of life, whatever such a notion might mean. It is a mistake, to put it mildly, to interpret libertarianism as a blueprint for life, a secular religion or philosophy that has a "solution" for all life problems. The dystopia of Ayn Rand's novels projects an individualist philosophy fit for some adults, but not for children or disabled adults. That is one of the reasons why her novels appealed, and continue to appeal, to healthy adolescents and young adults much more than they do to mature men and women or chronically ill persons.

Although libertarian principles were never supposed to apply to domestic relations, their non-applicability is sometimes construed as a deficiency. For example, in *Love & Economics*, gauchely subtitled, *Why the Laissez-Faire Family Doesn't Work*, Jennifer Roback Morse writes: "This deficiency in libertarianism is dramatized in the characters created by Ayn Rand, one of the most radical and consistent individualists of the twentieth century. Her heroes have no childhoods."[5] Morse is right. But who said that the "laissez-faire family" works?

The point is that the legal and political framework of a free society, fit for healthy adults, cannot be based on the needs of dependents and their relations to caretakers.[6] Kenneth Minogue makes this point eloquently: "The state is essentially an association of independent and resourceful individuals living under law and, from a political point of view, the poor and the needy are nothing less than a threat to our freedom. They are, for example, the materials of the demagogue, who tries to gain power by promising to use the coercive power of the state to redistribute benefits."[7]

These reflections explain why, as the state increasingly treats adults as patients, the language of traditional political philosophy atrophies, and instead we adopt the language of need-and-relief, disease-and-treatment for analyzing the relations of the citizen to the state. It is regrettable enough that we delegate to the state the care of individuals without family supports. It is folly to deliberately enlarge the scope of the state by adding fresh categories of claimants to its services.

In the past, we infantilized certain adults directly, typically women. Today, we do so indirectly, by treating them as if they were dependents, unable to survive without the "help" of the government. The template for this therapeutic dehumanization by infantilization may be summarized as follows:

> Anyone may be a victim of X. Having X transforms productive, law-abiding adults into unemployed, lawless quasi-children. Such persons pose a threat to themselves and others, hence must be protected from themselves and society must be protected from them. Proper help-therapy, that only agents of the state can provide, will turn such victims back into productive, law-abiding tax-payers, "saving money" for society's producers. Depriving the victims of X of liberty—often necessary for their rehabilitation—is not a deprivation of freedom; on the contrary, it is the guaranteeing of their right to liberation from the shackles of X.

In this formula, X may stand for drug addiction, mental illness, racial or gender status, poverty, child abuse, and so forth. The result is a steadily expanding roster of "liberation rights" and "therapy rights." At the same time, our elementary acts of self-determination—exemplified by self-medication and suicide—are treated as offenses against criminal and mental health laws, and our basic obligations as adults, to ourselves and others—exemplified by being held responsible for contracts and crimes—are abrogated by psychiatric excuses and tort litigations undreamed of a mere half a century ago.[8]

Property, the Foundation of Liberty

Since the publication of Smith's *Wealth of Nations* in 1776, it has become commonplace, especially among libertarians, to regard private property and individual liberty as two sides of the same coin. Mises developed this theme so fully that little needs to be added to it. "If one abolishes man's freedom to determine his own consumption," he wrote, "one has taken all freedom away."[9]

It was also clear, already in Smith's day, that the peaceful market offers a more effective means for raising peoples' material well being than do economic arrangements based on command and coercion by a centralized political authority (theocratic rulers, the totalitarian state). However, most peoples' need for personal security is greater than their need for material security. They crave to overcome the terrifying experience of feeling lost in a strange and threatening world—an experience that is universal in childhood and often persists into adulthood. That insecurity generates a yearning for dependence on a benevolent authority—God, great leaders, doctors, the state. Moreover, it is the lot of mankind to feel not only insecure but also bored. To combat that experience, people long to be passively entertained, which requires less effort than assuming responsibility for self-improvement.

In addition, vast numbers of adults are lazy, and want "bread and circuses." Since it is easier to destroy than to build, people find the spectacle of the destruction of life, liberty, and property endlessly entertaining, a truism in the light of the history of the species and its present use of television and war.

Honoring the values of industriousness, competence, and steadfastness requires a generosity of spirit and a curbing of envy, traits that not enough people esteem and fewer still cultivate and acquire. Not until "human nature" itself progresses morally will the majority of people prefer peaceful and boring market relations to the violent and exciting relations between coercer and coerced, predator and victim.

"Aid" and the Unchained War Metaphor

Until World War II, the American system of social controls rested on Christian moral values and was enforced by a judicial apparatus based on English common law, the Constitution, and the rule of law. Since then, our system of social controls has become increasingly dependent on the principles of a politicized medicine, and has been legitimized and enforced by a complex state apparatus that commingles the principles and practices of coercive psychiatry, collectivistic public health, and the criminal justice system. To articulate this insight, I proposed three new terms: "myth of mental illness," "therapeutic state," and "pharmacracy/ pharmacrat."

The term "myth of mental illness" (1960) is intended to indicate that neither unwanted behaviors nor psychiatric diagnoses are diseases.[10] "Therapeutic state" (1963) identifies the autocratic political system, legitimized by medical (especially psychiatric) symbols and interventions, that systematically subverts the protections of individual liberty guaranteed by the Bill of Rights and the rule of law.[11] The term "pharmacracy" (1974) refers to the use of medical (especially psychiatric) methods in the service of political rule and social control; "pharmacrats" are persons engaged in promoting and enforcing the principles and practices of pharmacracy.[12]

Coincidentally, Wilhelm Röpke identified the ideas and interventions of socialist economists in similar terms. He wrote: "The prototype of the modern economocrat is the eighteenth-century physiocrat. The physiocrats...are clearly the ancestors of all the power-thirsty, cocksure, and arrogant [economic] planners and organizers."[13]

The threats of economocracy and pharmacracy to individual liberty, personal responsibility, and the free society go hand in hand. The respective professionals and their hangers-on, especially in the media, are fanatic supporters of the tutelary state, seeking to expand government control over the daily lives of the citizenry by economic and medical interventions and regulations.[14] The clearest illustrations of the actual workings of economocracy and pharmacracy are foreign aid and psychiatric aid (usually called "mental health services" or "psychiatric services"). Both augment the power and wealth of the bureaucrats who distribute it, and exacerbate the miseries of the people they are supposed to benefit.

It is axiomatic, in debates about and the literature on foreign aid, that poverty is bad and prosperity is good. It does not seem to occur to people that this value system is inconsistent with the basic economic message of Christianity (and not only Christianity). Holiness is associated with poverty, not riches. The New Testament brims with homilies such as these:

Luke 1: 53: "He hath filled the hungry with good things; and the rich he hath sent away." 2 Corinthians 8: 9: "For ye know the grace of our Lord Jesus Christ, that, though he was rich, yet for your sakes he became poor, that ye through his poverty might be rich." And, most famously, Matthew 19: 23-24: "Then said Jesus unto his disciples, Verily I say unto you, that a rich man shall hardly enter into the kingdom of heaven. And again I say unto you, It is easier for a camel to go through the eye of a needle, than for a rich man to enter into the kingdom of God."

To be sure, Protestantism is a form of Christianity, and the celebrated Protestant ethic is often and rightly credited with advancing capitalism and prosperity. Protestantism, however, is called that for good reason: It was a *protest* against certain "fundamentalistic" Catholic principles and practices, from celibacy to usury.

The inchoate belief that being rich is somehow shameful or sinful has a long history, probably originating from a primitive fear of jealous gods. The Greek philosopher Isocrates (436-338 B.C.) complained: "One must now apologize for any success in business, as if it were a violation of the moral law, so that today it is worse to prosper than to be a criminal."[15] Helmut Schoeck, a German sociologist, attributed the modern version of this attitude to the role of envy in human affairs.[16] Peter Bauer (Lord Bauer), a Hungarian-British economist, characterized relations between First and Third World countries as ruled by "the economics of resentment."[17] I agree with these interpretations.

In an essay characteristic of the genre, Jeff Gates—co-founder and president of the Orwellian-titled Shared Capitalism Institute—urges the confiscation ("taxation") of astronomical sums from the rich and their redistribution among the poor. "The mission of the Shared Capitalism Institute," according to its website, is "to enhance the level of public debate about a long-neglected cause of fast-widening economic disparities both within and among nations: *non-inclusive patterns of ownership*."[18] Gates explains: "Political instability and terrorism are fueled by persistent and abject poverty and by fast-widening economic inequality both within and among nations."[19] Crime is due to mental illness, terrorism is due to poverty. The cures are clear: eliminate the enemies. In the case of poverty, the cure, according to Gates, is "inclusion," a code word for worldwide Marxist egalitarianism.

Gates sees the solution to the "problem of poverty" in various taxes, one of which he calls the "freeloader fee": "If the *geopolitical community coalesced* to identify the owners of an estimated 1.5 million tax haven accounts, up from 200,000 since the late 1980s, an *annual* 'freeloader fee' of 3.5 per cent could generate as much as $350 billion, assuming the amount in tax havens is in the mid-range of $10 trillion."

Gates is nothing if not inventive. He knows other people's secrets. By definition, deposits in tax havens are undisclosed. How, then, does he know that the number of such accounts grew more than seven-fold in less than twenty years? Facts and truths are irrelevant in his holy war against poverty—a war against a veritable "plague." Gates writes: "Persistent abject poverty should be viewed as *a modern-day plague, a paradigm-deficiency* that fuels the instability and terrorism that jeopardizes development."

Gates's discovery of the new disease, "paradigm-deficiency," is a medical breakthrough. Why, we might ask, should we view poverty as a disease, if it is not a disease? And if we view it as a disease, shouldn't we expect it to be fought by doctors? The Nazi image of the Jew as disease-spreading vermin here reappears unchanged, as Gates's anticapitalist image of the poverty-spreading rich. Gates continues: "Much like the multilateral effort to systematically *eradicate smallpox*, the geopolitical community has the financial and technical wherewithal to *identify and surround abject poverty until this age-old scourge* disappears from the anguished face of humankind. As part of that process, the dominant development model must be revised to promote inclusive development as a way to *inoculate against this disease's recurrence*."[20]

In Gates's "inclusive" new world, individuals have no right to own anything. Only the "geopolitical community" has such a right. Gates's mad logic leads him to a positively comical gloss on the glorious side-effects of his scheme of expropriation. Since the scale of confiscation and redistribution he envisions would be vast, it would require a huge army of bureaucrats to administer. This, in itself, would be an economic boon, as it would provide jobs to vast armies of unemployed: "As a logistical challenge, a worldwide War on Poverty is *a massively labor-intensive endeavor, akin to conventional war in the mobilization of human and financial capital required.* The jobs that such an effort would generate—in both the developed and the developing world—may be just the tonic required to recover from a fast-globalizing overcapacity that endangers economic recovery worldwide."[21]

Gates is not alone. Similar calls to arms abound. "Half the world's population lives on less than $2 a day," warns a report in the *Baltimore Sun*:

> A sixth of the population, more than 1 billion people, lives on less than a dollar a day.... People living on the margin are easy recruits for terrorism [like poor Osama bin Laden].... Picture the world as a large airliner. The Americans are reclining in first class, watching personal video screens, enjoying drinks and nuts.... The poor are huddled on the wings, some are clinging for their lives, others sawing off pieces to sell for scrap. The events of Sept. 11 have shown that we ignore the poor at our peril.... The poor are sawing the wings off the global airliner as we speak.[22]

The poor suffer from a plague. They get it from the rich, who are immune to it. The poor are airline passengers "huddled on the wings," sawing off their seats. It would be difficult to say whose bombasts and medical fantasies are more imaginative and impressive: those of the rhetoricians of foreign aid or of psychiatric aid?

The Rhetoric and Politics of "Aid"

The typical political-philosophical justification for the state is the need to protect the community from criminals at home and enemies abroad. The peace of the community is now believed to be threatened by two other groups as well: destitute people in underdeveloped countries, and mentally ill people in developed countries. Virtually across the political spectrum, people take for granted that caring for and coercing these persons is the duty of the governments of democratic-developed countries. It is this belief—in "need" on the one side, "duty to relieve" on the other—that defines these two dependent-dangerous classes, whose members have, in reality, little in common except for being regarded by others—richer and more powerful than themselves—as requiring economic assistance or psychiatric treatment.

In the course of the past thirty-five years, I devoted several books and essays to showing that in waging wars against drugs and mental diseases, the modern therapeutic state—exemplified by the United States—produces more of what it ostensibly wants less of. It creates more drug use, more drug trafficking, more dependency, more disability, and more crime, all attributed to drugs and mental illnesses. Along the way, it also creates more social controls, all labeled as "rights" and "treatments."

Although my criticism of mental health policy resembles the conservative-libertarian criticism of welfare policy, it has not received similar support. One reason for this may be the medical-therapeutic terminology of psychiatry that creates an utterly misleading image of the "problem." Accepting this usage precludes honest examination of the moral legitimacy of the psychiatric enterprise and dispassionate appraisal of the benefits and detriments of psychiatric coercions and excuses.[23]

While I was developing a systematic critique of mental health policy, Bauer was developing a systematic critique of foreign aid policy. The two critiques closely resemble one another. This is not surprising. The parallels between them are, in fact, present. And Bauer and I were good friends. Much of what Bauer says about foreign aid policy holds true for, and applies even more powerfully to, psychiatric aid policy, with this difference: libertarian economists oppose foreign aid, but there are no libertarian psychiatrists to oppose psychiatric slavery.

Parenthetically, I note here that some people call me a "libertarian psychiatrist," a label I prefer to the false label "antipsychiatrist." However, both labels miss important points. The label "anti-psychiatrist" is false, because I favor distinguishing between contractual and coercive psychiatry and oppose only the latter; hence, I do not consider myself an antipsychiatrist. However, distinguishing between contractual and coercive psychiatric practices is, in effect, illegal: everyone considered a psychiatrist is obligated to practice coercion. Hence, the term "libertarian psychiatrist" is an oxymoron.[24]

Bauer and I also agreed on the crucial role that the rhetoric of altruism and compassion plays in aid policies and in short-circuiting cogent debate about them. He wrote:

> To call official wealth transfers "aid" promotes an unquestioning attitude. It disarms criticism, obscures realities, and prejudges results. Who can be against aid to the less fortunate? The term has enabled aid supporters to claim a monopoly of compassion and to dismiss critics as lacking in understanding and compassion.... It is foreign aid which has brought into existence the Third World (also called the South) and which thus underlies the so-called North-South dialogue or confrontation. Foreign aid is the source of the North-South conflict, not its solution. Take away foreign aid, and there is no Third World or South as aggregate. A further pervasive consequence of aid has been to promote or exacerbate the politicization of life in aid-receiving countries.... An unquestioning attitude prevails in public discussion of this policy. Discussions on this subject in legislatures, especially in Europe, are not debates but are akin to seminars of like-minded aid supporters or enthusiasts.[25]

Foreign aid, Bauer pointed out, "is paid by governments to governments; it is not a redistribution of income between persons and families."[26] It is certainly not a form of assistance given by a donor to recipient. Instead, it is a payment by a government, American or European, to another government, ostensibly to help the needy. The actual result is that the intermediary—typically, an African despot—uses some of the funds to line his own pockets and the rest to purchase the goods and services necessary to subjugate and terrorize his people. The situation in the case of publicly funded psychiatric services is similar. The donors are the taxpayers. The recipients are psychiatric institutions and organizations, who use some of the funds to enrich their members and employees, and the rest to purchase the goods and services necessary to subjugate and frighten the denominated and would-be beneficiaries.

Bauer observed: "There are many examples from the experience of the last two decades of the comparative ineffectiveness of foreign aid as an instrument for raising the general living standards and promoting long-term economic development in poor countries."[27] In the case of psychiatry, the evidence is even more dramatic. The experience not of two decades but two centuries has demonstrated the utter ineffectiveness of public psychiatry in reducing the incidence or severity of the conditions psychiatrists call "mental diseases." I long ago concluded that, in such instances, we deal with symbolic-ceremonial policies, not with practical-technical policies, such as the provision of potable water or hygienic sewage disposal.[28]

Bauer scoffed at what he called "the axiomatic case for foreign aid"— "the unanimous opinion of all foreign-aid experts that the total amount of development aid is grossly inadequate for even the minimum needs of the developing countries.'"[29] If we replace the phrase "the unanimous opinion of all foreign-aid experts" with "the unanimous opinion of all psychiatric experts"; "the total amount of development aid" with "total amount of public funds spent on psychiatric services"; and "the minimum needs of the developing countries" with "the minimum needs of the mentally ill," we arrive at the axiomatic case for psychiatric aid. Not surprisingly, every respectable public organization, national and international, supports both foreign aid and psychiatric aid.

The two largest international organizations sponsoring and supporting foreign aid are the World Bank and the International Monetary Fund (IMF).[30] The World Bank represents a membership of 184 countries, with approximately 8,000 employees in Washington and "over 2,000 in the field." The Bank's website identifies the organization as "one of the world's largest sources of development assistance. Its primary focus is on helping the poorest people and the poorest countries.... Mission: Our dream is a world free of poverty." Regarding the scope of the World Bank's assistance programs, we read: "In 2002 the World Bank provided $19.5 billion to developing countries.... We live in a world so rich that global income is more than $31 trillion a year. In this world, the average person in some countries earns more than $40,000 a year. But in this same world, 2.8 billion people—more than half the people in developing countries—live on less than $700 a year. Of these, 1.2 billion earn less than $1 a day."[31]

Other sponsors of foreign aid are the United Nations (UN), the World Health Organization (WHO), and the governments of the western, donor countries. Psychiatric services are supported by a similar array of leading international and national organizations, among them the UN, WHO, World Federation for Mental Health (WFMH), United States government, National Institute for Mental Health, Supreme Court, ACLU, American Bar Association, American Medical Association, American Psychiatric Association, American Psychological Association, National Alliance for the Mentally Ill, international pharmaceutical industry, and many other mental health, anti-smoking, anti-obesity, anti-gambling, and other anti-sin and anti-crime lobbies. Opposing these mammoth charitable-therapeutic organizations—whose goals are chimerical and whose prestige is independent of the consequences of their actions—is a quixotic undertaking. The critic may be right, but this has nothing to do with the matter. The real, in contrast to the avowed, purpose of both foreign aid and psychiatric aid is to enhance the donors' self-esteem and keep the unwashed and unwanted away from the door.[32]

In a salute to Bauer shortly before his death, *The Economist* cited his mordantly witty definition of foreign aid as "an excellent method for transferring money from poor people in rich countries to rich people in poor countries."[33] *Mutatis mutandis*, providing government-funded mental health services is an excellent method for transferring money from relatively poor taxpayers to relatively rich psychiatrists and other practitioners of psychiatric-psychological disablement.

After decades of neglect, Bauer's views gained a measure of support among libertarian and conservative economists and politicians.[34] Still, it is important to recognize that the forces he was up against are similar to the forces a critic of psychiatric services is up against, and that these forces continue to gain strength.

Economics and Psychiatry: What are They Really About?

The parallels between foreign aid and psychiatric aid are but one facet of the similarities between economics and psychiatry. Another, more basic, facet is that neither economics nor psychiatry is about what the leaders of these disciplines say they are about: the former is not about mathematics or finance, and the latter is not about diseases of the brain or psychopharmacology. James Buchanan's views are especially relevant and useful in this connection.

Buchanan, a Nobel Laureate in Economics, says what he means and says it clearly. He asserts that the very term "economics" is misleading. "I should propose that we cease, forthwith, to talk about *economics* or *political economy*, although the latter is the much superior term. Were it possible to wipe the slate clear, I should recommend that we take up a wholly different term such as *catallactics*, or *symbiotics*.... [The term "symbiotics"] conveys, more or less precisely, the idea that should be central to our discipline...attention to a unique sort of relationship, that which involves the cooperation of individuals, one with another, even when their individual interests are different."[35] Conversely, the idea central to psychiatry is conflict and non-cooperation, that is, conflict within the "patient" and between him and other individuals and institutions (laws). (The term "catallactics" has not caught on, perhaps because people are reluctant to face its antonym and call it by its rightful name, "*coercetics*," a term that fits regulatory economics loosely, and psychiatric slavery perfectly.)

Cooperative human relationships are, of course, not unique to economics. What is unique is that, according to Buchanan, these relationships ought to form the principal or sole subject matter of economics. This perspective is consistent with Adam Smith's seminal concept of the "invisible hand." Buchanan illustrates his point with the example of Robinson Crusoe. Alone on his island, Crusoe makes choices, but his choices are *not economic choices*; they become economic choices only after he begins to cooperate with Friday. Similarly, I have emphasized that, as long as Crusoe is alone, he could have malaria, but could not have schizophrenia. Why not? Because malaria is the name of a parasitic disease that could well kill him, whereas schizophrenia is the name of a behavior that connotes conflict. Crusoe could "develop" schizophrenia only after he and Friday come into conflict and Friday so labels Crusoe's behavior. "Mental illness," qua psychiatric diagnosis, is the products of *conflict between persons*.

"The market or market organization," Buchanan emphasizes, "is not a means toward the accomplishment of anything. It is, instead, *the institutional embodiment of the voluntary exchange processes* that are entered into by individuals in their several capacities. This is all there is to it."[36] Contrariwise, psychiatry is *the institutional embodiment of the coercive relationships* that are imposed upon individuals in their several capacities as psychiatric physicians and mental patients. Psychiatry is not a means toward the accomplishment of helping, treating, or curing; it is social control.

With exceptional clarity, Buchanan explains: "Insofar as individuals exchange, trade, as freely contracting units, the predominant characteristic of their behavior is 'economic.'... Insofar as individuals meet one another in a relationship of superior-inferior, leader to follower, principal to agent, the predominant characteristic of their relationship is 'political.'... Economics is the study of the whole system of exchange relationships. *Politics is the study of the whole system of coercive or potentially coercive relationships.*"[37] For many years, the term "psychiatry" denoted two wholly different, mutually incompatible enterprises: voluntary psychiatry and involuntary psychiatry, one based on exchange between equals, the other based on domination and subjection between superiors and inferiors. As I noted earlier, psychiatry based on contract and exchange is now tantamount to medical negligence.[38]

Emphasizing that economics deals with choice, Buchanan approvingly cites Robert Mundell's definition of it as "the science of choice" and adds: "I propose to examine this assertion seriously and critically.... I want to ask whether a *science of choice* is possible at all. Are we not involved in a contradiction in terms?"[39] Buchanan answers this question with a resounding yes: "Choice, by its nature, cannot be predetermined and remain choice. If we then define science in the modern sense of embodying conceptually refutable predictions, a 'science of choice' becomes self-contradictory."[40] A science of coercion is a self-contradiction not only because we cannot make verifiable predictions about its consequences, but because science rests on cooperation and is incompatible with coercion.

Buchanan urges economists to "stay within the exchange paradigm," and considers measuring "social costs and social benefits" exercises in economic scientism.[41] He writes: "[L]et us recall here that Professor Tjallings Koopmans won a Nobel Prize in economics, not in engineering. He did so for his efforts that commenced from working out the optimal allocation of a set of tankers plying oil across the Atlantic during World War II, where the variables were ships, distances, port locations, barrels of oil, and, of course, a set of shadow prices."[42] Concluding, Buchanan warns:

Economics seems unlikely to escape from this chaos for many years, if indeed it survives at all as an independent discipline.... For myself, I advance no claim that my own thinking has yet fully rid itself of the paradigms of neoclassical orthodoxy.... I am tempted to emulate Hayek and entitle this postscript essay, "Why I Am Not an Economist." To anyone who reads the methodological urgings contained in the essays in this volume...and who simultaneously looks at what passes for "economics" in the professional journals of 1980, there is only one evident conclusion. The author of the essays is almost the only one in step or else writes under some delusion that he is something that he is not.[43]

The Jacobins, observed Burke, having unmoored themselves from the restraints of custom and moderation, "have found their punishment in their success."[44] The same fate may befall economists and psychiatrists.

The Naked Emperors

Economists and psychiatrists have vested interests in mystifying their activities. They make economics and psychiatry appear to be subjects at once recondite and indispensable for society, scholarly disciplines whose principles and practices ordinary people cannot understand without many years of academic study. This is not true. It requires no academic degree to recognize that industriousness is more likely to contribute to material well-being than idleness, that modesty and self-discipline are more conducive to an orderly life than conceit and spitefulness.

It is not an accident that when economists look at economic behavior, they tend to see something wrong that needs fixing: unemployment, industrial activity, interest rates, the trade deficit or surplus are too high or too low; people save/spend too much or too little. Similarly, when psychiatrists look at human behavior, they also tend to see something wrong that needs fixing: mania and depression; overactivity and underactivity; people eating too much or too little, having too much interest in sex or not enough. The result is that economics and psychiatry both provide a rationale for remedying problematic (unwanted) behaviors, and a justification for using the coercive apparatus of the state to accomplish that end.

The principal economic aim of the government thus becomes titrating the precise interventions needed to make the economic system function optimally—a "healthy economy" as a steadily expanding economy. The Federal Reserve System intervenes with its particular remedial tools—"jawboning," issuing bonds, raising or lowering interest rates—to fine-tune the economy.

The principal psychiatric aim of the government becomes a similar process of micromanagement, titrating the precise interventions needed to make the social system function optimally—a "mentally healthy nation" as a nation free of drug abuse, crime, and mental illness. The psychiatric system intervenes with its particular therapeutic tools—diagnoses, drugs, and coercions—to fine-tune the lives of human beings and the "mental health" of the community.

Economic and psychiatric remedies are parts of the problems. The free market is supposed to be self-regulating. However, it can be said to be "free" only in so far as it is allowed to be self-regulating. The same is true for a free adult in a modern, secular society with limited government. The citizen is supposed to be self-regulating, yet he can be said to be "free" only in so far as he is allowed to be self-regulating. This is why libertarians oppose, and must oppose, state monopoly of the issuing of money (legal tender), a point emphasized by both Hayek and Rothbard. For the same reason, libertarians must oppose the state's toleration of psychiatric coercions and recognition of psychiatric excuses.

As matters stand, politicians, pundits, and the public "know" that underdeveloped countries need foreign aid and cannot develop without it. In 2002, U.N. Secretary General Kofi Annan declared: "[M]any [poor countries] are saying that in order to make the full transition to sound, open economies, they need increased aid from wealthier countries."[45] Bauer liked to point out that, at one time, developed countries too were underdeveloped. How did they become developed and rich without foreign aid? If they could do it, he insisted, so could others, provided they adopt the proper economic, legal, and political measures.

Similarly, politicians, pundits, and the public "know" that children suffering from oppositional-defiant disorder and other mental disorders need psychiatric help and cannot develop without it. In fact, the idea that children have "mental disorders" that require psychiatric treatment is a very recent invention. Prior to the twentieth century, there was no child psychiatry and there were no such diseases. Yet, not only did children—even "deprived" children—manage to grow up and live productive and successful lives, they did so causing much less trouble to parents and society than they do now.

There is no mystery about the ingredients needed to secure a free government, economic development, or personal competence. "To make a government," observed Burke, "requires no great prudence. Settle the seat of power; teach obedience; and the work is done. To give freedom is still more easy. It is not necessary to guide; it only requires to let go the rein. But to form a *free government*; that is, to temper together these opposite elements of liberty and restraint in one consistent work, requires much thought; deep reflection; a sagacious, powerful, and combining mind."[46]

The recipes for economic and personal development are similar. Both require individuals who want to improve their lot here on earth rather than in heaven, and are willing to learn, work hard, and cooperate with others. They also require that when people come together in society, they create laws to protect private property, tolerate a significant measure of economic inequality, and form a government whose exactions do not discourage the accumulation of capital. Education, training, machinery, and technological innovation are additional stimuli to economic growth, each person's prosperity subtly aiding every other person's. "It is in the interest of the commercial world," said Burke, "that wealth should be found everywhere."[47]

It is easier to define prosperity than sanity. Nevertheless, I venture to suggest, without pursuing the matter here, that similar considerations hold true for achieving what people regard as a state of mental health or, better, avoiding a state of mental illness. To paraphrase Burke, it is in the interest of both a prosperous and a "sane" world that learning, reflection, self-reliance, and liberty-with-responsibility be found everywhere.

Among the forces that retard economic development (prosperity) and personal development (mental health) are political oppression, paternalistic social policies, and excessive interest in God and religion—and, from our present interest most importantly, "helping" individuals capable of helping themselves and having the duty to do so.

Reconsidering Liberty and Psychiatry

Defined broadly, freedom is an ancient concept, as the Biblical story of the Exodus illustrates.[48] *The libertarian idea of individual liberty as freedom from arbitrary coercion by the state* is relatively new—a product of the Reformation, the Enlightenment, secularism, individualism, limited government, and the free market. *The "progressive" idea of freedom as therapeutic liberation by oppression* is newer still.[49]

Economically, the lot of mankind throughout most of history was poverty; politically, it was subjection to despotism; and intellectually, it was abject ignorance. For a small, educated minority, freedom was a spiritual concept—mastery of the passions and submission to the will of God. In the sixteenth century, the condition of people in Western Europe began to undergo a radical transformation. I shall summarize some of the signposts along the road that man has traveled in his quest for *personal independence*, a journey that is still in its early stages.

- •   1517: Martin Luther (1483-1546) publishes *Disputation on the Power and Efficacy of Indulgences*, signaling the beginning of what we know as the Reformation. Especially in its Calvinist incarnation, the Protestant ethic and the spirit of capitalism (Max Weber) provides sanction for replacing preoccupation with religion with disciplined work: the study of nature, improvement of living conditions, and accumulation of wealth.

- •   1531: Henry VIII (1491-1547) becomes the supreme head of the Church of England, beginning England's emancipation from the papacy. A century and a half later (1687), Isaac Newton (1642-1727) publishes the *Mathematical Principles of Natural Philosophy* (*Philosophiae Naturalis Principia Mathematica*), ushering in the modern age, based on science.

- •   1690: John Locke (1632-1704) publishes *Essay Concerning Human Understanding* and *Two Treatises of Government*.[50] In these works— which had the profoundest influence on the Founders—Locke establishes the principles of modern empiricism and lays down the doctrine that government rests on popular consent, its powers are limited, and rebellion is permissible when government subverts its just and proper ends—protection of life, liberty, and property. "Good and evil, reward and punishment, are the only motives to a rational creature: these are the spur and reins whereby all mankind are set on work, and guided."[51]

- •   1776: Adam Smith (1723-1790) publishes *An Inquiry into the Nature and Causes of the Wealth of Nations*, and the United States declares its independence from Britain (*The Declaration of Independence*).

These developments in moral and political thought have remained unequaled to the present. We have since concentrated on science and made giant strides in biology, chemistry, and physics, a progress that threatens the moral values and political fabric of our civilization. The utopian promises of science debauched into scientism encourage politicians and the people to ignore *the limitations of government to do good, and of science to explain human behavior and correct human misbehavior.*

Conclusion

"Democracies," James Madison (1751-1836) warned: "have ever been spectacles of turbulence and contention; have ever been found incompatible with personal security or the rights of property; and have in general been as short in their lives as they have been violent in their death."[52] The Founders did not create a democracy. The time may yet come when we wake up and realize that democracy is inimical to liberty and responsibility.

Like other critics of the French Revolution, Sir Henry Sumner Maine (1822-1888), the great nineteenth-century historian and legal scholar, regarded the masses as deficient in self-responsibility and hence unfit for popular government. "Democracy," he declared, "is commonly described as having an inherent superiority over every other form of government.... It is thought to be full of the promise of blessings to mankind; yet if it fails to bring with it these blessings, or even proves to be prolific of the heaviest calamities, it is not held to deserve condemnation. These are the familiar marks of a theory which claims to be independent of experience and observations."[53]

Nevertheless, Maine remained optimistic about the possibilities of moral evolution. In *Ancient Law*, his best-known work (cited briefly in the Preface), he offered this important historical observation:

> The movement of the progressive societies has been uniform in one respect. Through all its course it has been distinguished by the gradual dissolution of family dependency and the growth of *individual obligation* in its place.... The advance has been accomplished at varying rates of celerity.... But, whatever its pace, the change has not been subject to reaction or recoil, and apparent retardations will be found to have been occasioned through the absorption of archaic ideas and customs from some entirely foreign source. Nor is it difficult to see what the tie between man and man which replaces by degrees those forms of reciprocity in rights and duties which have their origin in the Family. *It is Contract*. Starting, as from one terminus of history, from a condition of society in which all the relations of Persons are summed up in the relations of Family, we seem to have steadily moved towards a phase of social order in which all these relations arise from the free agreement of individuals. In Western Europe the progress achieved in this direction has been considerable. Thus the *status of the Slave has disappeared—it has been superseded by the contractual relation of the servant to his master*. The status of the Female under Tutelage, if the tutelage be understood of persons other than her husband, has also ceased to exist; from her coming of age to her marriage all the relations she may form are relations of contract.... The apparent exceptions are exceptions of that stamp which illustrate the rule. The child before years of discretion, the orphan under guardianship, *the adjudged lunatic*, have all their capacities and incapacities regulated by the Law of Persons. But why? The reason is differently expressed in the conventional language of different systems, but in substance it is stated to the same effect by all. The great majority of Jurists are constant to the principle that the classes of persons just mentioned are subject to extrinsic control on the single ground that they do not possess the faculty of forming a judgment on their own interests; in other words, that they are wanting in the first essential of an engagement by Contract. The word Status may be usefully employed to construct a formula expressing the law of progress thus indicated...*we may say that the movement of the progressive societies has hitherto been a movement from Status to Contract*.[54]

Let us follow Maine and take the long view. For thousands of years, man regarded work as a curse and prosperity as a sin, a perspective supported by the New Testament. Only in recent memory, only in some parts of the world, and only for some people did work become a blessing and property a virtue. I submit that the development of the Protestant ethic was, in fact, a first step toward what we ought to call the atheist ethic. Maine, as I noted, stated: "...we may say that the movement of the progressive societies has hitherto been a *movement from Status to Contract*." *Pari passu*, the movement of the progressive societies has been a *movement from Theism to Atheism.*

The great monotheistic religions came into being as ethical aids. As people replace faith with reason, a God that punishes and forgives becomes an ethical impediment not only to socially broadly based material progress, but to the widespread assumption of personal responsibility. Unfortunately, many people continue to use religion in this way and also embrace its secular-"humanist" twin, psychiatry, as an added aid in this evasion.

In the history of the twentieth century, the principal *dramatis personae* were National and International Socialisms, better known as Nazism and Communism. Their citizens evaded the duty of self-responsibility by claiming to be "following orders." Following orders—attributed to or issued by God, the State, Science, Medicine—is always the easy way out. Refusing to do so requires self-reliance and resisting temptations and threats.

In what promises to be the history of the twenty-first century, the principal *dramatis persona* left on the historical stage is the Home of the Free, better known as the United States. Its citizens evade the duty of self-responsibility by claiming to be the helpless victims of temptations and traumas. Refusing to do so requires thinking for oneself and resisting the enticements of the blame-game and the profits of legal predation justified by the principle of *caveat vendor.*

The challenges of modernity—particularly individual liberty and personal responsibility—will not go away. The escapes from responsibility offered by religion, totalitarianism, and psychiatry are likely to be but temporary setbacks in humanity's moral evolution. We are at the beginning, not the end, of the history of man as moral agent.

II

Profiles:

Where Some Famous Libertarians Went Wrong

A. Civil Libertarians

5

John Stuart Mill

The name of John Stuart Mill (1806-1873) is, or ought to be, familiar to every educated person. There is a vast literature on his life and work, on which I shall touch only in so far as it is relevant to the theme of my book.

Mill's father, James Mill (1773-1836), was the son of a Scottish cobbler. A self-made man, he created a meteoric career for himself as philosopher, educator, and man of letters. He married Harriet Burrow, whose mother—Mill's grandmother—"kept an asylum for lunatics in Hoxton."[1]

Unlike many of his famous contemporaries, John Stuart Mill had no inherited wealth and had to make a living by working. In his *Autobiography*, Mill tells us: "In May, 1823, my professional occupation and status for the next thirty-five years of my life, were decided by my father's obtaining for me an appointment from the East India Company, in the Office of the Examiner of India Correspondence, immediately under himself."[2] It is reasonable to assume that these circumstances contributed to his paternalistic attitude toward colonial people, and antipaternalistic attitude toward persons we call "users of illegal drugs," but who in Mill's time were users of legal products.

The East India Company was the commercial flagship of British colonialism. One of its principal sources of revenue was the opium trade. The Mills—both father and son—were, in current parlance, employees of the greatest drug cartel of all times. This occupation happened to be consistent with their utilitarian ideology. After all, there is probably no more direct and effective method for facilitating "the greatest happiness for the greatest number" than by giving people access to opium in the free market.

Mad-doctoring and *On Liberty*

By the time Mill began to address the conflict between psychiatric incarceration and individual liberty, the English people were familiar with the subject, often sensationalized in the popular press. As early as 1728, Daniel Defoe (1661-1731), the famed author of *Robinson Crusoe*, denounced what we now call "psychiatric abuses." He wrote:

> This leads me to exclaim against the vile Practice now so much in vogue among the better Sort, as they are called, but the worst sort in fact, namely, the sending their Wives to Mad-Houses at every Whim or Dislike, that they may be more secure and undisturb'd in their Debaucheries: Which wicked Custom is got such a Head, that the number of private Mad-Houses in and about London, are considerably increased within these few Years. This is the height of Barbarity and Injustice in a Christian Country, it is a clandestine Inquisition, nay worse.[3]

In 1858, a year before publishing *On Liberty*, Mill criticized what later became known as "false commitment." In a letter to the London *Daily News*, he warned:

> Sir,—It has become urgently necessary that public attention should be called to the state of the law on the subject of Lunacy and the frightful facility with which any persons whom their heirs or connections desire to put out of the way, may be consigned without trial to a fate more cruel and hopeless than the most rigorous imprisonment.... The obvious remedy is to require the same guarantees [as for imprisonment for crime] before depriving a fellow-creature of liberty on one pretext as on another. The inquiry by a jury, which is now the exception, ought to be the rule.... Juries, in such cases, are foolish and credulous enough, and only too willing to treat any conduct as madness which is ever so little out of the common way; but at least the publicity of the inquiry is some protection, and tends to fix attention on any unavowed motive which may actuate the promoters of the proceeding.... I earnestly intreat you to continue your efforts at rousing public opinion on a matter so vital to the freedom and security of the subject.[4]

Mill did not oppose psychiatric imprisonment, as such. He opposed only the laxity of the procedures used to implement the "lunacy laws." Mill's statement, "Juries...[are] only too willing to treat any conduct as madness which is ever so little out of the common way," implies that if the conduct is "out of the common way" more than "ever so little," then it may justify the use of psychiatric segregation. Here begins the descent down the slippery slope. Once we grant power to medical agents of the state to coerce innocent persons—in the name of undefined and undefinable "dangers" to themselves or others—there is no practical way to prevent them, and their social superiors, from "abusing" the law.

On Liberty is one of the most famous books in the literature of political philosophy generally, and of libertarianism in particular. The views Mill expresses in it have far-reaching implications on all our policies toward all so-called victimless crimes. Its implications on psychiatric practices are less obvious, but no less relevant. In this book, Mill famously declared:

> Over himself, over his own body and mind, the individual is sovereign. It is, perhaps, hardly necessary to say that this doctrine is meant to apply only to human beings in the maturity of their faculties. We are not speaking of children.... Those who are still in a state to require being taken care of by others, must be protected against their own actions as well as against external injury. For the same reason, we must leave out of consideration those backward states of society in which the race itself may be considered as in its nonage.... Despotism is a legitimate mode of government in dealing with barbarians, provided the end be their improvement, and the means justified by actually effecting that end.[5]

Without saying whether insane persons are fit or unfit for political freedom, Mill added this prescient warning: *"Each [person] is the proper guardian of his own health, whether bodily, or mental and spiritual.* Mankind are greater gainers by suffering each other to live as seems good to themselves, than by compelling each to live as seems good to the rest."[6] Few people then shared this view, and even fewer share it today. According to today's conventional wisdom, a person diagnosed as mentally ill is not the proper guardian of his own health, wealth, or anything else.

Mill continued: "The only part of the conduct of anyone, for which he is amenable to society, is that which concerns others. In the part which merely concerns himself, his independence is, of right, absolute. Over himself, over his own body and mind, the individual is sovereign."[7] Mill called behaviors that concern only the self "self-regarding," and behaviors that concern others as well "other-regarding." Although people disagree about where to draw the line between these two classes of actions, the distinction remains one of the guiding principles of the free society. Although rarely phrased in these terms, one of the most important political questions that faces us is: Which acts concern the actor only and thus fall outside the scope of legislative control, and which concern the public as well and are properly the business of the state?

Acts generally considered self-regarding range from reading books to practicing religion, rights guaranteed by the First Amendment. Some may grant self-regarding status also to certain behaviors that are potentially or actually self-destructive, such as hang-gliding, skydiving, and suicide. Acts generally considered other-regarding range from creating a public disturbance to crimes such as driving while intoxicated, assault, and murder. Overeating, drinking alcohol to excess, and smoking cigarettes, marijuana, or opium in private exemplify acts that some people regard as self-regarding and others as other-regarding. In this respect, another point needs to be emphasized. For example, masturbation in private is self-regarding, while heterosexual coitus, especially if it results in pro-creation, is clearly other-regarding. Yet, it does not follow that it ought to be subject to regulation by the state, much less prohibited by it.

Since the latter half of the nineteenth century, the ideology of public health and psychiatry together with socialist politics have endeavored to erase the differences between the interests of the self and interests of society, between injuring oneself and injuring others. "Every injury to the health of the individual is, so far as it goes, a public injury," declared English philosopher Thomas Hill Green (1836-1882).[8] With this dictum as their creed, health statists—led by the mental health lobby—have largely succeeded in convincing Americans that such radically different behaviors as killing oneself and killing others are similar: each is a manifestation and/or consequence of mental illness. The result is a negation of the differences between dangerousness to self and dangerousness to others: the private sphere, free of state regulation, merges into the public sphere, the object of state regulation. The professionals charged with destroying the differences between self- and other-regarding behaviors and coercing troublesome persons—some of whom are guilty of breaking the law, and most of whom are not—are psychiatrists, in Mill's day called "mad-doc-tors." Mill denounced their work with these scathing words:

> But the man, and still more the woman, who can be accused either of doing "what nobody does," or of not doing "what everybody does," is the subject of as much depreciatory remark as if he or she had committed some grave moral delinquency.... [F]or whoever allow themselves much of that indulgence, incur the risk of something worse than disparaging speeches—they are in peril of a commission *de lunatico*, and of having their property taken from them and given to their relatives.... There is something both contemptible and frightful in the sort of evidence on which, of late years, *any person* can be declared judicially unfit for the management of his affairs; and after his death, his disposal of his property can be set aside, if there is enough of it to pay the expenses of litigation.... These trials speak volumes as to the state of feeling and opinion among the vulgar with regard to human liberty.... In former days, when it was proposed to burn atheists, charitable people used to suggest putting them in a madhouse instead; it would be nothing surprising now-a-days were we to see this done.[9]

Although *On Liberty* is a short book, Mill used it to state and restate his commitment to the adult person's right to self-determination, even if it entails self-harm:

> But neither one person, nor any number of persons, is warranted in saying to another human creature of ripe years, that he shall not do with his life for his own benefit what he chooses to do with it.... Considerations to aid his judgment, exhortations to strengthen his will, may be offered to him, even obtruded on him, by others: but he himself is the final judge. All errors which he is likely to commit against advice and warning are far outweighed by the evil of allowing others to constrain him in what they deem his good.... Acts injurious to others require a totally different treatment.... The distinction between the loss of consideration which a person may rightly incur by defect of prudence or of personal dignity, and the reprobation which is due to him for an offense against the rights of others, is not a merely nominal distinction.[10]

Mill's following remarks are even more timely today than they were when he offered them, 150 years ago:

> If protection against themselves is confessedly due to children and persons under age, is society not equally bound to afford it to persons of mature years who are equally incapable of self-government? If gambling, or drunkenness, or incontinence, or idleness, or uncleanliness, are as injurious to happiness, and as great a hindrance to improvement, as many or most of the acts prohibited by law, why (it may be asked), should not law, so far as is consistent with practicality and social convenience, endeavor to repress these also?... I fully admit that the mischief which a person does to himself may seriously affect, both through their sympathies and their interests, those nearly connected with him and, in a minor degree society.... No person ought to be punished simply for being drunk; but a soldier or a policeman should be punished for being drunk on duty.[11]

Why did Mill believe that adults should have such a far-reaching right to self-determination? Because he viewed children as the prisoners (my metaphor, not his) of society:

> Society has had absolute power over them during all the early portion of their existence: it had the whole period of childhood and nonage in which to try whether it could make them capable of rational conduct in life.... If society lets any considerable numbers grow up mere children, incapable of being acted on by rational considerations of distant motives, society has itself to blame for the consequences.... [I]t is not difficult to show, by abundant instances, that to extend the bounds of what may be called moral police, until it encroaches on the most unquestionably legitimate liberty of the individual, is one of the most universal of all human propensities.[12]

What do children, slaves, serfs, mental patients, and persons living in totalitarian states have in common? Their "personal lives" are not their own. Mill continued:

[L]eaving people to themselves is always better, *ceteris paribus*, than controlling them...there are questions relating to interference with trade which are essentially questions of liberty: such as the Maine Law [prohibiting alcohol in that state in the U.S.]...*the prohibition of the importation of opium into China; the restriction on the sale of poisons; all cases, in short, where the object of interference is to make it impossible or difficult to obtain a difficult commodity. These interferences are objectionable, not as infringements on the liberty of the producer or seller, but on that of the buyer.... [As for the dangerousness of drugs]...he ought, I conceive, to be only warned of the danger, not forcibly prevented from exposing himself to it...*the buyer cannot wish not to know that the thing he possesses has poisonous qualities. But to require in all cases the certificate of a medical practitioner would make it sometimes impossible, always expensive, to obtain the article for legitimate uses.... If people must be allowed, in whatever concerns only themselves, to act as seems best to themselves, at their own peril, they must equally be free to consult with one another about what is fit to be so done; to exchange opinions, and give and receive suggestions.[13]

Mill's views on drug controls are even more timely now than they were in his day: "When we compare the strange respect of mankind for liberty, with their strange want of respect for it, we might imagine that a man had an indispensable right to do harm to others, and no right at all to please himself without giving pain to any one."[14]

Are Mental Patients Like Minors?

In all societies, children and adults occupy different social spheres. In advanced societies, the difference is institutionalized in the form of a distinct legal role and status for each. In the modern West, adults are presumed to be legally competent and responsible for their actions. They cannot be coerced by agents of the state for their own good, but can be as punishment for crimes. With children, the opposite is the case. Children are presumed to be legally incompetent and not responsible for their actions. They can be coerced by agents of the state for their own good, but cannot be punished the same way adults can be.

These distinctions are fundamental to Mill's philosophy. He used the term "nonage," now obsolete, to designate persons who, regardless of their chronological age, have not yet reached, or perhaps will never reach, maturity. He believed that such persons were rightfully treated as if they were minors. The idea of insanity (madness, mental illness, psychiatric disorder), as I have shown, combines and conflates the ideas of illness, incompetence, irresponsibility, and nonage.[15] Mental illness is a strategic fiction. People called "mentally ill" ought to be treated as responsible adults. Psychiatric coercions constitute paradigmatic violations of the rule of law and are incompatible with the principles that ostensibly distinguish "free" from "unfree" societies.

During the Middle Ages, only persons whose behavior resembled the behavior of "wild beasts" were categorized as insane. In the eighteenth century, after the trade in lunacy became established, the category of insanity began to expand and the traditional bracketing of the insane with infants and idiots as proper subjects of coercion by relatives and the state became increasingly useful and acceptable, both socially and legally.

From 1823 until 1858, Mill was an officer in the East India Company. His statement, "we must leave out of consideration those backward states of society in which the race itself may be considered as in its nonage," was a defense of English colonial policy in India, whether or not it was so intended. This concession greatly weakened his argument about liberty in general, and especially about liberty for persons whose mental powers did not measure up to some unspecified minimum standard. If it was proper to coerce the "immature" members of "backward races," it was also proper to coerce the "immature" members of advanced races, called "mental patients."

Sir James Fitzjames Stephen (1829-1894), in his celebrated critique of Mill's *On Liberty*, recognized the Achilles heel in Mill's remark and properly attacked him on that vulnerable point:

> You admit that children and human beings in "backward states of society" may be coerced for their own good.... Why then may not educated men coerce the ignorant?... It seems to me quite impossible to stop short of this principle if compulsion in the case of children and "backward" races is admitted to be justifiable; for, after all, maturity and civilization are matters of degree. One person may be more mature at fifteen than another at thirty.[16]

Stephen was right. Mill's argument is valid only if his premise is valid, that is, only if insane adults resemble children so significantly that it is legitimate to subject them to "benevolent" rather than "punitive" coercion. This premise is patently invalid. Yet, the facile bracketing of "infants, idiots, and insane," combined with the pretense that psychiatric imprisonment is treatment not punishment, has long justified, and continues to justify, psychiatric slavery. "Freedom," writes Milton Friedman, "is a tenable objective only for responsible individuals. We do not believe in freedom for madmen or children."[17] This aside illustrates the enduring power of the image of "the insane" as a dependent infant in need of care, incompetent to know his own interests.

The differences between a child and a mental patient are embarrassingly obvious. The criterion for minority is objective: chronological age. The criterion for mental illness is not merely not objective, it is nonexistent. Psychiatric diagnosis is an inference that often rests on absurd criteria. For example, the presence of mental illness may be inferred from the subject's place of residence and history: if he resides in a mental hospital or has a history of mental hospitalization, he may be identified as mentally ill on that ground alone.

The so-called "psychiatric examination"—ostensibly to determine whether a person suspected of being mentally ill is in fact mentally ill—is a charade, mimicking the medical examination. What evidence of "illness" does the psychiatrist look for? He looks for deviant, socially prohibited ideas, feelings, or behaviors, exemplified by "delusions" and "hallucinations."

Perhaps most important are the glaring differences between infants and the insane with respect to their respective capacities for doing serious mischief to others and for taking care of themselves if need be. Infants do not shoot presidents or commit suicide. The so-called insane do. Deprived of caretakers, infants perish, while most insane persons survive and often become indistinguishable from sane persons. This is what enables insane persons, but not infants, to survive on the streets and disturb the social order. In sum, bracketing insanity with infancy—placing persons diagnosed as mentally ill in the same class as persons considered of "nonage"—is not based on evidence. It is a legal strategy that serves important social interests.[18]

None of this means that I deny that many "neurotics" are "infantile," a point both Freud and Jung emphasized. However, infantilism of one sort or another is a universal human trait. Moreover, it is one thing to say that a five-year-old who wets his pants is "immature," and quite another to say that a twenty-five-year-old who joins a cult and spends his time worshiping his guru is immature. One man's immaturity is another man's religiosity.

In any case, an attribution of childishness lends no support to the medical concept of mental illness and cannot justify the juridical-philosophical claim that the law ought to treat adults called "mental patients" *as if* they were children. Existential immaturity—regardless of how we define or identify it—is not a brain disease. A childish adult needs to grow up, not be treated with drugs by doctors or with detention by judges. Let us not forget that, in the past, the argument that blacks and women were child-like was used to deprive them of rights and responsibilities. Today, the same argument is used to deprive mental patients of rights and responsibilities.

Utilitarianism and the Problem of Happiness

Before concluding this chapter, a few words need to be said about utilitarianism. Early in his essay on the subject, Mill offered this definition: "The creed which accepts as the foundation of morals, Utility, or the Greatest Happiness Principle, holds that actions are right in proportion as they tend to promote happiness, wrong as they tend to produce the reverse of happiness. By happiness is intended pleasure, and the absence of pain; by unhappiness, pain, and the privation of pleasure."[19]

Utilitarianism is a modernized and sanitized kind of Christianity. Or, as Mill put it: "If it be a true belief that God desires, above all things, the happiness of his creatures, and that this was his purpose in their creation, utility is not only not a godless doctrine, but more profoundly religious than any other."[20] And again: "In the golden rule of Jesus of Nazareth we read the complete spirit of the ethics of utility. To do so as you would be done by, and to love your neighbor as yourself, constitute the ideal perfection of utilitarian morality."[21] (Matthew 7:12 and Luke 6:31: "All things whatsoever ye would that men should do to you, do ye even so to them: for this is the law and the prophets.")

In a recent study of Mill's "religion," Linda Raeder cogently concludes that although Mill adhered, in part, to the principles of classical liberalism, he

> muddied the waters of classical liberal philosophy and practice with his conviction that the end of government is the all-encompassing "improvement of mankind" and not the preservation of individual liberty under law, as well as with his self-conscious embrace of the "social"-ist moral ideal.... The result of this attempt was the curious and unstable hybrid of modern liberalism, which attempts to promote the socialist moral ideal of collective service to humanity through expansive, activist government and this in the name of the very individual freedom that classical liberalism was concerned to secure.... Mill's refusal to recognize the connection between human freedom and the imperfection of existence is, however, quite consistent with his frequent demands for a visible and transparent "social justice," that Trojan horse of Anglo-American collectivism.... Mill, in perhaps his most important incarnation, is the first modern liberal.[22]

Mill was also, in a sense, the first modern pharmacrat. Samuel Johnson was right: Hell *is* paved with good intentions. Perhaps the single greatest obstacle to a decent and free society is *obsession with making other people happy*, whether they like it or not.

The fallacy of utilitarianism, like the fallacy of psychiatry, rests on and is inherent in its terminology. Treating Happiness as if were a "thing" that can exist in the aggregate is nonsense. The term "happiness" denotes a wholly subjective mental state and can predicate only persons. *Collectivities cannot be happy*. To be sure, groups of people can be free of pain or suffering—for example, of the suffering associated with high infant mortality or an epidemic of tuberculosis. But improvements in human health in the aggregate have not made people happy; they have made them covetous of a life free of disease and pain and even death.

In the end, *Mill's utilitarian ethic offers tempting justification for the initiation of psychiatric violence.* In the modern world, the subjection of the weak to the strong is regularly justified by the rhetoric of protection and "treatment." Mill is deservedly famous for his struggle against the legal inequality between women and men, and hence the subjection of the former to the latter.[23] It is all the more surprising, then, that he endorsed other, unspecified kinds of legal inequalities: "All persons are deemed to have a right to equality of treatment, except when some recognized social expediency requires the reverse."[24]

Conclusion

Mill's head was libertarian, but his heart was utilitarian. He could never shake off the belief system he inherited from his father, James, and their intellectual patron, Bentham.

Having said that, Mill deserves our admiration and respect, not least for the moral grandeur of his character. That grandeur, in combination with his intellect, allowed him to be hopeful about human progress—not as the continuous increase in the quantity of "human happiness," but rather as the intermittent but steady diminution of political oppression. Near the end of *Utilitarianism*, Mill observed:

> The entire history of social improvement has been a series of transitions, by which one custom or institution after another, from being a supposed primary necessity of social existence, has passed into the rank of a universally stigmatized injustice and tyranny. So it has been with the distinctions between slaves and freemen, nobles and serfs, patricians and plebeians; and so it will be, and in part already is, with the aristocracies of color, race, and sex.[25]

And so, I believe, it will be with the distinction between the mentally ill and the mentally healthy. Psychiatric slavery, too, shall "pass into the rank of a universally stigmatized injustice and tyranny." This, too, will not make people happy, but it will make them more free and more responsible.

6

Bertrand Russell

Bertrand Arthur Russell (1872-1970)—the third Earl Russell, scion of one of the oldest and noblest families in England, mathematician, philosopher, political activist, lecturer, Nobel laureate in literature—was the preeminent celebrity intellectual of the twentieth century.

Russell was not a libertarian. However, as the *Encyclopaedia Britannica* acknowledges, his "eloquent championing of individual liberty... made his position in the intellectual life of his time comparable with that of Voltaire in the 18th century or with that of J. S. Mill in the 19th."[1]

Because Russell professed to be interested in freedom and espoused "progressive" views about crime, education, marriage, and heterosexual (though not homosexual) relations, he is, mistakenly, often considered a libertarian. In fact, he was the very opposite, a utopian-therapeutic socialist, resembling Rousseau and Robespierre, rather than Voltaire or Mill.

Russell's childhood began tragically and was unhappy. His mother, Lady Alderley (1842-1874), daughter of Lord Stanley, died when he was two; his father, John Russell (Lord Amberley, 1842-1876), died when he was four. Orphaned at an early age, Russell was raised by his paternal grandparents, Lady Frances Anna Maria Elliot Russell (Countess Russell, 1814-1898), and her husband, Lord John Russell (Earl Russell, 1792-1878). Thanks to his natural gifts, noble parentage, superior education, and zest for knowledge and intellectual work, Bertrand Russell became one of the most brilliant men of his age.

However, the experience of ordinary family happiness was denied him. "In adolescence," he recalled, "I hated life and was continually on the verge of suicide, from which, however, I was restrained by the desire to know more mathematics."[2] His own odd and unhappy childhood may have contributed to his inability, despite his apparent best efforts, to create a satisfactory family life for his children. In 1930—when his son, John, was nine years old, and his daughter, Kate, seven—Russell wrote rhapsodically: "For my own part, speaking personally, I have found the happiness of parenthood greater than any other that I have experienced."[3] He spoke too soon. Before long, parenthood became the greatest source of unhappiness in his life.

Roads to Freedom

In the vast opus of Russell's published works, perhaps none provides better insight into his character than does *Roads to Freedom*, a book he wrote in 1918, before entering prison for objecting to the war.[4] Subtitled, *Socialism, Anarchism, and Syndicalism*, the book is a long sermon on egalitarianism, socialism, and the "therapeutic" approach to crime and punishment.

"What," asks Russell, "is the fundamental evil in our modern Society which we should act to abolish?" He answers: "Poverty is the symptom: slavery the disease."[5] Note the medical metaphor. Before considering Russell's views about psychiatry, some of his other ideas about the good society are worth noting.

- Education should be compulsory up to the age of sixteen.... When education is finished, no one should be *compelled* to work, and those who choose not to work should receive a bare livelihood, and be left completely free.[6] (Thirty-three years later, Russell wrote: "So great is this evil that the world would be a better place, at any rate, in my opinion, if State education had never been inaugurated."[7])

- The expense of children will not fall, as at present, on the parents. They will receive, like adults, their share of necessaries, and their education will be free.[8]

- Marriage should be a free, spontaneous meeting of mutual instinct, filled with happiness not unmixed with a feeling akin to awe.[9]

- At present a very large part of the criminal law is concerned in safe-guarding the rights of property, that is to say—as things are now—the unjust privileges of the rich.[10]

- There will not be the capitalist management, as at present, but management by selected representatives.... Payment will not be made, as at present, only for work actually required and performed, but for willingness to work.[11]

Anticipating the writings of Franz Alexander and Karl Menninger on crime and psychiatry, Russell declared:

The more we study the question [of crime], the more we are brought to the conclusion that society itself is responsible for the anti-social deeds perpetrated in its midst, and that no punishment, no prisons, and no hangmen can diminish the number of such deeds; nothing short of a reorganization of society itself.... When a man is suffering from an infectious disease, he is a danger to the community, and it is necessary to restrict his liberty of movement.... The same method in spirit ought to be shown in the treatment of what is called "crime."[12]

At the earliest light of the dawning therapeutic state, Russell naively embraced the psychiatric perspective on crime and punishment:

The first thing to recognize is that the whole conception of guilt or sin should be utterly swept away.... [T]he important thing is to prevent the crime, not to make the criminal suffer. Any suffering which may be entailed by the process of prevention ought to be regarded as regrettable, like the pain involved in a surgical operation. The man who commits a crime from an impulse to violence ought to be subjected to a *scientific psychological treatment*, designed to elicit more beneficial impulses.... It may also be conceded that impulses toward criminal violence could be very largely eliminated by a better education. But...we cannot suppose that there would be no lunatics in an Anarchist community, and *some of these lunatics would, no doubt, be homicidal*. Probably no one would argue that they ought to be left at liberty.... Those who nevertheless still do commit crimes will not be blamed or regarded as wicked: they will be regarded as unfortunate, and kept in *some kind of mental hospital until it is thought that they are no longer a danger*.... By the method of individual *curative treatment*, it will generally be possible to secure that a man's first offence shall also be his last, except in some cases of *lunatics and the feeble-minded, for whom a course of more prolonged but not less kindly detention may be necessary*.[13]

Russell's views on crime, punishment, and therapy presage the views of contemporary psychiatrists and policy analysts, both liberal and conservative. I have criticized these ideas and interventions elsewhere.[14]

Power and Psychiatry

Russell was an exceptionally well-informed man. He had studied the works of James B. Watson and Sigmund Freud, admired them as scientific psychologists, fancied himself a keen psychologist, and offered many pronouncements about matters we regard as falling in the province of the anthropologist, psychologist, and psychiatrist. For example:

- The Chinese are gentle, urbane, seeking only justice and freedom.[15]

- It seems on the whole fair to regard negroes as on the average inferior to white men.... Women are on the average stupider than men.... One can generally tell whether a man is a clever man or a fool by the shape of his head.[16]

Like his contemporaries, Russell entertained a special interest in eugenics. He wrote: "The sterilization of the unfit is within the scope of immediate practical politics in England. The objections to such a measure...are, I believe, not justified. Feeble-minded women, as everyone knows, are apt to have enormous numbers of illegitimate children, all, as a rule, wholly worthless to the community. *These women would themselves be happier if they were sterilized.*"[17] By "unfit," Russell meant persons suffering from mental deficiency and mental illness or "insanity." Note that Russell imputed happiness to women sterilized against their will.

Who should determine whether a person is "unfit"? Russell believed this is a task for psychiatrists. Lamenting Russell's "faith in psychiatric definitions and diagnoses," Ray Monk, his biographer, observes that Russell "did not regard mentally ill people as having any value to society or of deserving any rights or consideration. As far as he was concerned, to become insane was virtually to lose one's status as a person."[18] *Mutatis mutandis*, to be *declared* insane was, and is, to lose one's status as a person. That, precisely, was Russell's attitude toward his son, John, whom he treated as an insane nonperson.

Russell was well aware that the work of the psychiatrist differs radically from the work of the regular physician. The psychiatrist has no markers for the alleged diseases he diagnoses and treats. The involuntary mental patient—*the only kind that existed during Russell's formative years*—regards his psychiatrist as his adversary, not ally.

Sprinkled through Russell's writings are indications that he was cognizant of the true nature of the phenomena psychiatrists and people generally label "mental illnesses." Instead of mental illness, Russell used the term "insanity." For example, in *The Conquest of Happiness* (1930)—a hodgepodge of platitudes, obtuse bigotries, and perceptive observations—Russell wrote: "In its more extreme forms persecution mania is a recognized form of insanity.... This, like many other forms of insanity, is only an exaggeration of a tendency not at all uncommon among people who count as normal. I do not propose to discuss the extreme forms, which are a matter for a psychiatrist."[19]

Russell correctly identifies "paranoid" suspiciousness as an exaggerated form of normal human behavior, a "tendency." In the next sentence, he washes his hands of it, asserting that only a psychiatrist—that is, a medical doctor—is competent to deal with it. But Russell full well knew the difference between unwanted human behavior and pathological alteration of the human body. How does exaggerated suspiciousness become a disease? What is insanity? Why should insane persons be deprived of liberty? Despite all his brilliance and erudition, Russell never asked himself these questions. All his life, he claimed to be fighting for individuals and groups deprived of liberty by the holders of power, yet wanted to subject persons he viewed as insane to the despotic powers of psychiatrists.

In his book *Power* (1938), Russell presented an astute analysis of the megalomania intrinsic to madness as a manifestation of the subject's unsatisfied thirst for power. He wrote:

> The love of power is a part of normal human nature.... The existence of the external world, both that of matter and that of other human beings, is a datum, which may be humiliating to a certain kind of pride, but can only be denied by a madman. *Men who allow their love of power to give them a distorted view of the world are to be found in every asylum: one man will think he is the Governor of the Bank of England, another will think he is the King, and yet another will think he is God. Highly similar delusions, if expressed by educated men in obscure language, lead to professorships of philosophy; and if expressed by emotional men in eloquent language, lead to dictatorships.* CERTIFIED lunatics are shut up because of their proneness to violence when their pretensions are questioned; the UNCERTIFIED variety are given the control of powerful armies, and can inflict death and disaster upon all sane men within their reach. The success of insanity, in literature, in philosophy, and in politics, is one of the peculiarities of our age, and the successful form of insanity proceeds almost entirely from impulses towards power.[20]

I agree with Russell's foregoing analysis, but of course reject his view that "shutting up certified lunatics" is justice or good social policy. Russell interpreted, I think correctly, the lunatic's behavior as goal-directed, and just as rational, subjectively speaking, as the behavior of the philosopher or the politician. In my view, what follows is that the criminal behavior of "lunatics" be controlled by the same laws that we use to control the criminal behavior of non-lunatics.

Russell's use of the English locution "shut up" to mean "lock up" or "incarcerate" deserves a brief comment. When used to refer to "shutting up" mad persons, the term has at least three distinct meanings, each important, namely: 1) preventing the subject from speaking or refusing to listen to him; 2) refusing to understand what he tells us, misinterpreting his message by translating it into the idiom of psychiatry or psychoanalysis; treating his speech as if it were a pathological specimen, like sputum, not as a human communication of distress, or conceit, or a combination of them;[21] and 3) literally shutting up—that is, imprisoning—the subject. The relatives of persons who call on psychiatrists to incarcerate their "loved ones" and the psychiatrists who do the incarcerating engage in all three kinds of shutting up of the "patient."[22] In *Power*, Russell perceptively observed:

> While animals are content with existence and reproduction, men desire also to expand, and their desires in this respect are limited only by what imagination suggests as possible. *Every man would like to be God, if it were possible; some few find it difficult to admit the impossibility.* These are the men framed after the model of Milton's Satan, combining, like him, nobility with impiety. By "impiety" I mean something not dependent upon theological beliefs: *I mean refusal to admit the limitations of individual human power....* It is this that makes social cooperation difficult, for each of us would like to conceive of it after the pattern of the cooperation between God and His worshipers, with ourself in the place of God. Hence competition, the need of compromise and government, the impulse to rebellion, with instability and periodic violence. And hence the need of morality to restrain anarchic self-assertion.[23]

Clearly, Russell here sees madness in existential, not medical, terms, which makes his enthusiasm for psychiatric incarceration inconsistent with his zealous defense of individual liberty against other encroachments.

Bertrand Russell vs. John Russell

In 1921, when Russell was forty-nine years old, he and his second wife, Dora Black, had a son, John. Two years later, they had a daughter, Kate. Russell said he adored his children and wanted them to grow up in an atmosphere best suited for their development. To this end, he created a school devoted to creating "a generation educated in fearless freedom.... If existing knowledge were used and tested methods applied, we could, in a generation, produce a population almost wholly free from disease, malevolence, and stupidity. We do not do so because we prefer oppression and war."[24]

Believing that the root of much evil in the world stems from egoism (the rest he attributed to capitalism and poverty), Russell was determined to prevent his children from becoming egotistical. The worst thing for a child, Russell believed, was to think of himself "as the center of the universe.... A child is on the whole better fighting with other children than being coddled by grown-up people."[25] Accordingly, in the school he and his wife operated, the teachers' foremost duty was to treat all students alike. In practice, this meant that the Russell children, to prove the absence of favoritism toward them, were treated worse than other children. Denying his own elephantine egoism, Russell equated loyalty to one's own children—that is, favoring them over other peoples' children—with coddling them. "Show your love for your child by not showing it," he advised in his book, *On Education*.[26]

According to Kate's recollections, the school years were "an almost unmitigated misfortune," especially for John: "Not only was he bullied by the other children, but he also, in a sense, lost his parents, who were reluctant to appear to be favoring him in front of the other pupils, leaving him feeling abandoned and hurt.... I do not see how John endured it as he did...."[27] The answer is that John endured Russell's style of upbringing at the cost of never really growing up.

Bertrand Russell craved intimate human relations, yet also dreaded and avoided them as restraints on his freedom. Thrice divorced, he acted as if loyalty to wife and children were bad habits to be avoided at all cost. Kate managed to grow up. John, however, remained a child, an unwanted adult dependent, whom his father despised and defined as mad. Russell maintained that John was a "homicidal lunatic" who ought to be permanently confined in an insane asylum. Actually, he was a pathetic, passive person who never displayed any physical aggression toward anyone. It was Russell who was psychiatrically homicidal toward him.

From 1938 until 1944, the Russells lived in the United States. Russell taught at prestigious universities and enjoyed lucrative tours as a popular lecturer. John attended Harvard, drifted to California, adopted an openly homosexual lifestyle, and neither held a real job nor earned any real money. Back in England with his parents after the war, he became emotionally as well as economically dependent on them. By this time, Dora Black and Bertrand Russell had been unamicably divorced and both had remarried. John's fate became an important bone of contention between them. Russell was determined to psychiatrically dispose of John. Dora tried to save him from Russell and psychiatry. Ray Monk documents this horrifying tale so thoroughly that some critics have scorned his work as unfairly harsh towards Russell. However, the evidence Monk assembles leaves no doubt that Russell had an irrational fear of John and, for his own security, felt that John should be locked up.

John's psychiatric saga began in earnest in 1954, when—unemployed and unhinged—he went to see his daughters who were in Russell's care. "Russell, alarmed at his mental state, arranged for his own doctor, Dr. Boyd, and a psychiatrist called Desmond O'Neill to come and remove John to the psychiatric ward at Guy's Hospital, where he was diagnosed as suffering from a 'serious state of delusional insanity' and given insulin to induce him into a coma.... To have his son go insane was the realization

of Russell's very deepest fears."[28] In the spring of 1955, "John was incarcerated in no fewer than three different psychiatric institutions," each
time at his father's instigation.[29]

Monk writes: "Russell was determined to leave the care of John in
the hands of medical authorities and have as little to do with him as possible," while his mother, Dora, wanted to care for him.[30] In May 1955,
realizing at long last that his father was waging a psychiatric war against
him, John prepared a psychiatric will that stated:[31] "To all whom it may
concern: During my illness I wish my mother Mrs. Dora Winifred Grace
of the above address to be consulted and to have authority to deal with
my affairs and matters relating to me and my children. John Russell."[32]

Relations between Dora and Russell were so bad that they commu-
nicated only through lawyers. Illustrative of Dora's desperate efforts to
save John from Russell's determination to "shut him up" is her letter to
Louis Tyler, her solicitor: "And please do not take this matter lightly, but
try to get hold of his father at the earliest possible moment. In such a case
as John's, when he feels that he *has lost everything, that he is unwanted
and uncared for, the cure does not lie solely with chemistry or even with
psychiatry.*"[33] Dora recognized what ailed her son, but it was too late.

Neither John's psychiatric will nor Dora's efforts was a match for
Russell's resolve to see his son certified as incurably insane. Ironically,
John was saved from permanent psychiatric incarceration only by the
conscientiousness and decency of the psychiatrists who happened to be
in charge of determining his fate:

> [In July 1955,] Dora received a telephone call from John, telling her that
> doctors had arrived...to serve a committal order on him and that he therefore
> had no choice but to return to Holloway Sanatorium. This new Emergency
> Order gave Russell another seven days in which to get John certified, and he
> did not waste any time. His petition for John's certification was heard before
> a magistrate at a rapidly convened Board of Control meeting at Holloway
> Sanatorium on 7 July, the day before John's order expired.... Dora knew noth-
> ing about it until the afternoon of 7 July, when she phoned the sanatorium
> and was told that the question of John's certification was about to be decided.
> She at once took a taxi to Virginia Water, but arrived too late to attend the
> meeting and was shown into a waiting room to await the verdict. Presently,
> the magistrate, two members of the Board and a doctor came into the room
> to tell Dora that the petition had been unsuccessful. The decision reached
> was that...[John] was not certifiable.[34]

Russell remained unconvinced. Nine years later, Russell, now ninety-
two years old, was still trying to convince psychiatrists that John ought to

be incarcerated in a madhouse. Once again, he turned to a "Dr. Morgan" (who had examined John in 1957) to examine John and certify him as needing to be confined. "On 15 May [1964], Dr. Morgan submitted his report to the court. John, he wrote, far from getting worse, 'has improved enormously since I first saw him in 1957 and now needs no medication whatsoever.'"[35]

In 1970, Russell died and John succeeded him as Earl Russell. John Russell then "became a regular attender of—and occasional participant in—debates in the House of Lords, but he never fully regained his sanity. He died in 1987."[36]

Why did Russell torture his son by relentless efforts to secure his psychiatric imprisonment? Although my answer is speculative, I believe we must locate the explanation in the two paired emotions typically and most intensely generated in the family, namely, love-hate, and pride-embarrassment. Russell was proud of being an aristocrat and a celebrated intellectual. He wanted to be proud of his children: as we saw, he deliberately set out to make them into superchildren. Having failed dismally to accomplish this task, he concluded that he had produced infrachildren, hopelessly damaged by the hereditary madness affecting the Russell family. I am convinced that Monk is right, that Russell's snobbish vanity "is also, one suspects, at the root of his desire to have John certified [as permanently insane]. That the title of 'Earl Russell' might one day be inherited by a lunatic filled him with dread."[37]

Russell was deeply disappointed in, and embarrassed by, his son. As is often the case in such situations, the son denied the father's rejection and sought futilely the paternal respect and love that were not to be granted. The father had fame and money; the son had nothing. If such a father wants to separate himself from his grown son, he has two options. One option is to "divorce" the son; that is, let him swim or sink. The other is to define him as mentally ill and try to "dispose" of him as a mental patient permanently confined in an insane asylum. Russell knew all this. So why did he—why do so many parents—prefer to dispose of their young-adult children as mad rather than divorce them as unwanted? The answer is obvious and painful. Divorce leaves the son free to embarrass the parent, precisely what the parent wants to avoid; it also leaves the parent open to censure by kin and friends for "abandoning" his own child. Psychiatric disposition protects the parent at the expense of the child. The masks of "diagnosis" and "treatment" conceal the true nature of both problem and the solution. It effects the separation of father from son that the feather desires; at the same time, it casts the parent in the role of tragic victim, afflicted with a defective child for whom he "cares" with the medical treatment science has to offer. Russell was much too vain, self-centered, and angry at John to let him alone, even when Dora offered to take him out of Russell's hair.

Russell's "Horror of Madness"

Russell, Monk tells us, and meticulously documents, had a "horror of madness." What did he think "madness" was? Where did he get his ideas about what it was? I think he got them from the Zeitgeist of his age, from the misinformation he received from his grandmother, and from his own imagination.

The modern concept of madness is a creation of the post-Enlightenment mind and the social institutions developed for the control of individuals categorized as insane.[38] Russell grew up during the latter half of the nineteenth century. The concept of insanity to which he was exposed consisted of two main elements: the madhouse, symbolizing the incarceration of the mad person as an individual unfit to live in society, and "irrational" violence, symbolized by the image of the "homicidal lunatic."

The theme of the homicidal madwoman locked in the attic is the centerpiece of Charlotte Bronte's (1816-1855) famous novel, *Jane Eyre* (1847). Another nineteenth-century classic, *Frankenstein: The Modern Prometheus* (1818), by Mary Wollstonecraft Shelley (1797-1851)—daughter of the famed feminist Mary Wollstonecraft and the respected philosopher William Godwin—features a mad scientist and the out-of-control, homicidal, quasi-human being he created. Neither least nor last, there was *The Strange Case of Dr. Jekyll and Mr. Hyde* (1886), by Robert Louis Stevenson (1850-1894) that, perhaps more than any other single work of literature, fixed in the public mind the idea that madness and murder went hand in hand and were, indeed, essentially synonymous concepts. Also on this list belongs *The Island of Doctor Moreau* (1896), by H. G. Wells (1866-1946), a science-fiction fantasy featuring still another mad scientist who transforms animals into quasi-human monsters.[39] Each of these works taps into the uncanniness and dread of the mad person as someone not fully human, unpredictable, and dangerous. I assume that Russell was familiar with these works and that they contributed to his fantasies about and fears of madness.

In addition to such literary influences, Russell had to be aware of the momentous influence of the idea of insanity on English law in the nineteenth century, especially during its initial decades. The celebrated trial of Daniel McNaghten took place in 1843. McNaghten, a Scotsman, felt persecuted by the prime minister, Sir Robert Peel, and set out to kill him, but by mistake killed Peel's private secretary instead. McNaghten made no attempt to escape and did not deny his crime. To avoid hanging the defendant, the judge in effect directed the jury to declare him "not guilty by reason of insanity." McNaghten spent the remaining twenty-one years of his life incarcerated at Broadmoor, the first "hospital" for the criminally insane in the western world.[40] The McNaghten trial and its aftermath signaled the beginnings of a "medical-therapeutic" approach to crime and punishment.

Three more sources for Russell's ideas about insanity remain to be noted. One is the then dominant psychiatric doctrine that insanity is hereditary, that is, ancestors deemed to have been mad predispose—even doom—their descendants to madness. Another is "masturbatory insanity," the favorite psychiatric fantasy of nineteenth-century mad-doctoring: when insanity was not hereditary, it was due to "self-abuse."[41] Masturbation was then believed to be both a cause and a symptom of mental illness, just as now chemical imbalance in the brain is believed to be the cause of schizophrenia and bipolar illness, and forcible administration of neuroleptic drugs is considered an effective treatment for these alleged maladies.

Finally, Russell's grandmother, who raised her prematurely orphaned grandson, contributed to his ideas about madness. Before his first marriage, this woman, according to Monk, "revealed to him the extent of inherited madness in the Russell family.... 'Ever since, but not before, [Russell wrote in his *Autobiography*], I have been subject to violent nightmares in which I dream that I am being murdered, usually by a lunatic.'"[42] In fact, reprising the dramatic theme of *Jane Eyre*, Russell says that he began to dream "that his grandparents had deceived him, that his mother was not dead, but mad and hidden away in an asylum."[43]

In Russell's mind, the most important elements in mad-doctoring were incarceration, secrecy, and hypocrisy. These elements were, in turn, connected, in both the press and the popular mind, with the problem of so-called "false commitment," that is, relatives disposing of unwanted family members by having them committed, with the connivance of corrupt psychiatrists, to madhouses.[44]

The Evil Pair: Madman and Psychiatrist

Although Russell's views on insanity were based, in part, on the bizarre fantasy of the madman as partly human, partly beast, his understanding of psychiatry was basically accurate.

The image of a being half-human and half-animal is intrinsic to mythology. In the ancient world, people believed in the sphinx, a mythical, threatening figure, with the head and bust of a woman, and the body of a lion with wings. In the modern world, people believe in beings who appear to be goal-directed human beings but are in fact "dangerous lunatics," bereft of free will and criminal responsibility; and in a legal-psychiatric system whose proper function is to confine such persons in insane asylums, ostensibly for "treatment," but actually for the convenience of inconvenienced family members.

Apparently unable to rid himself of the mystical elements of madness, Russell continued, throughout his long life, to entertain inchoate fears of both the madman and the mad-doctor. The madman was a combination between a wild beast bereft of reason and a homicidal maniac single-mindedly driven to commit seemingly senseless murders. Similarly, the mad-doctor was a power-hungry, evil genius, obsessed with driving his hapless victims to destruction and death. In short, Russell believed in the mythology of mental illness and feared madness and madmen. At the same time, he recognized institutional psychiatry as a legal-social mechanism for controlling recalcitrant members of the family and had contempt for the psychiatrist as an evil figure.[45]

When Russell was in his eighties, he turned his pen to writing short stories. Five of these were published under the title *Satan in the Suburbs* in 1953.[46] In the Preface, Russell characterized his motive for this undertaking as cathartic: "To attempt a new departure at the age of eighty is perhaps unusual, though not unprecedented.... For some reason entirely unknown to me I suddenly wished to write the stories in this volume, although I had never before thought of doing such a thing. I am incapable of critical judgment in this field, and I do not know whether the stories have any value. All I know is that it gave me pleasure to write them...."[47]

The lead story, "Satan in the suburbs," is a crude parody of the psychiatrist (medical psychoanalyst, medical psychotherapist) as a demonic character whose treatment consists of arousing the destructive and self-destructive impulses lurking in the souls of his clients who then come to a terrible end. One patient kills himself, another ruins himself by a needless act of embezzlement, and still another, a Mrs. Ellerker, is "falsely" committed to an insane asylum.

Mr. Ellerker is an outstanding scientist, Mr. Quantox his less talented colleague. Dr. Murdoch Mallako is the psychiatrist. As a result of a scheme by Quantox and Mallako, Ellerker is ruined and kills himself. When Mrs. Ellerker accuses Quantox of complicity in ruining her husband, she is deprived of her voice: "An eminent psychiatrist was summoned, and agreed at once that poor Mrs. Ellerker's mind had become unhinged. Mr. Quantox was too valuable a public servant to be at the mercy of a hysterical woman, and Mrs. Ellerker, after being duly certified, was removed to an asylum."[48]

The narrator—a neighbor of Dr. Mallako—grows suspicious of the doctor's role in the patients' perdition. Toward the end of the story, he visits Mallako and confronts him with his suspicions. Instead of denying his part in the tragic end of his patients, Dr. Mallako boasts about it. Russell puts these words in his mouth:

> You imagine in your miserable way that you hate mankind. But there is a thousand times more hate in my little fingers than in your whole body. The flame of hate that burns within me would shrivel you to ashes in a moment. You have not the strength, the endurance, the will to live with such hate as mine.... You have not realized (how indeed should you, having an imagination of so paltry a scope?), you have not realized that revenge is the guiding motive of my life— revenge not against this man or that, but against the whole vile race to which I have the misfortune to belong. Very early in my life I conceived this purpose.[49]

Whereupon the narrator pulls out a gun, shoots Mallako dead, wipes off his fingerprints, and places the weapon in the dead man's hands. "For some time after putting an end to Dr. Mallako, I felt happy and carefree." The narrator, a decent and conscientious man, becomes depressed and is haunted by Dr. Mallako in his sleep. He meets "an intelligent and charming lady, who at first captured my attention by her knowledge of the more devious paths of psychiatry. Here, I thought, is someone who, should the need ever arise, as, please God, it will not, will be able to follow the strange convolutions of evil thought which it has been my misfortune to thread my way."[50] He marries the woman, but continues to feel anxious, acts distracted, and finally, after waking from still another nightmare, confesses the murder to his wife:

> "I killed Dr. Mallako," I told her. "You may have thought that you had married a humdrum scientific worker, but it is not so.... I killed Dr. Mallako, and I am proud of it!"

"There, there," said my wife, "hadn't you better go back to sleep?"

I raged and stormed, but my raging and storming were of no avail.... As morning came I hear her go to the telephone.

Now, looking out of my window, I see on the doorstep two policemen, and an eminent psychiatrist whom I have long known. I see the same fate awaits me as that from which I failed to save Mrs. Ellerker. Nothing stretches before me but long dreary years of solitude and misunderstanding....[51]

If we ignore or are ignorant of the chronology of Russell's life, we would be tempted to interpret this story as an effort at catharsis, Russell trying to purge himself of guilt for subjecting his son to psychiatric misunderstanding, misinterpretation, and mistreatment. However, *Satan in the Suburbs* was published *a year before* Russell began to use psychiatrists to persecute his son.

Russell also saw through the pretensions of the psychoanalysts. In his essay "The psycho-analyst's nightmare: Adjustment—a fugue" (1954), he portrayed analysts as abject agents of adjustment. Dr. Bombasticus—the author's stand-in for Freud—psychoanalyzes Hamlet, Lear, Macbeth, Othello, Antony, and Romeo, reducing their glorious conflicts to silly, unjustified hang-ups about their parents. At the end, realizing his misdeeds, Dr. Bombasticus cries out: "I am in Hell! I repent! I killed your souls."[52]

Did Russell, the great skeptic—who respected no "unproven" claims—really believe in the mythology of mental illness or did he merely use institutional psychiatry as a convenient legal-social mechanism for controlling recalcitrant members of his family? His representation of psychiatry in *Satan in the Suburbs* leaves us in no doubt about the answer. By 1953, and most likely for some time before—perhaps most of his life—Russell had no illusions about the true role of the psychiatrist and the mental hospital: he recognized the mad-doctor as an unscrupulous agent of social control and the asylum as a prison.

Conclusion: Russell, Apostle of Reason

From his earliest years, Russell's overriding passion was Reason. In his Introduction to *Sceptical Essays* (1928), he declared: "I wish to propose for the reader's favorable consideration a doctrine which may, I fear, appear wildly paradoxical and subversive. The doctrine in question is this: that it is undesirable to believe a proposition when there is no ground whatever for supposing it true."[53]

A fanatic rationalist and self-declared atheist and skeptic, Russell placed his faith in redeeming mankind by logic, rationality, and science.

As this god failed him, he gave up on the idea of saving mankind and switched to believing it deserved to be destroyed. Russell expressed this sentiment in "The Infra-redioscope," a poorly executed futuristic fantasy.[54] With the United States and the Soviet Union poised to destroy one another and all mankind, the fear of an imaginary invasion by Martians unites them:

> Before the hatching of the plot, East and West had been on the verge of war, and it was thought by many that the human race would exterminate itself in futile fury. Now, from fear of a wholly imaginary danger, the real danger existed no longer. The Kremlin and the White House, united in hatred of the wholly imaginary Martians, had become the best of friends.... "Perhaps," so ran his [the narrator's] meditations, "perhaps it is only through lies that men can be induced to live sensibly. Perhaps human passions are such that to the end of time truth will be dangerous. *Perhaps I have erred in giving my allegiance to truth....*"[55]

The story ends when the imaginary Martians turn out to be real and humanity is exterminated: "The machines fell silent. Universal death spread throughout the world. The Martians *had* come." A Martian historian, commissioned by the leader to record the last days of mankind, writes:

> That great Martian, having observed here and there among his subjects a somewhat weak-kneed sentimentality as regards those mendacious bipeds whom his hosts so gallantly and so deservedly exterminated, decided in his wisdom that all the resources of erudition should be employed to portray with exact faithfulness the circumstances preceding this victorious campaign. For he is of the opinion—and I am sure that every reader of the foregoing pages will agree with him—that it could not be a good thing to allow such creatures to continue to pollute our fair cosmos.... Every true Martian heart must breathe more freely now in the knowledge that these creatures are no more.[56]

In the trajectory of Russell's life, we can trace the transformation of a young man full of zeal for reason and liberty, yet with a soul corrupted by an excess of vanity and self-love, into an old man full of hatred for mankind. At the end of the next story, titled "The Guardians of Parnassus," Russell puts these words in the narrator's mouth: "*I have not known the joys of love, but I have known the joys of hate; and who shall say which are the greater?*"[57]

7

The American Civil Liberties Union

The National Civil Liberties Union (NCLU) was founded in 1917, by Roger Baldwin, Crystal Eastman, and Norman Thomas. Baldwin was a sociology teacher turned socialist activist, Eastman a labor lawyer and socialist journalist. Thomas was a Presbyterian minister turned social worker and, for many years, the standard-bearer and presidential candidate of the Socialist Party of America. In 1920, the NCLU was re-formed as the American Civil Liberties Union (ACLU), with Baldwin as its first president. Until the Hitler-Stalin pact of 1939, Baldwin was a staunch defender of the Soviet Union.

The ACLU claims to be the premier American organization for the protection of civil liberties. It does not claim to be a libertarian organization. In fact, it is an organization that promotes left-liberal, socialist political "reforms." Nevertheless, because of its name and reputation, a brief review of the ideas this influential group has put forth and the positions it has taken with respect to psychiatric principles and practices deserves to be included in this study.

The ACLU web site characterizes the nature and aims of the organization as follows:

> Since our founding in 1920, the nonprofit, nonpartisan ACLU has grown from a room-full of civil liberties activists to an organization of nearly 300,000 members and supporters, with offices in almost every state. The ACLU's mission is to fight civil liberties violations wherever and whenever they occur.....
>
> Three Things to Know About the ACLU:
>
> • We're for traditional American values. In many ways, the ACLU is the nation's most conservative organization. Our job is to conserve America's original civic values—the Constitution and the Bill of Rights—and defend the rights of every man, woman and child in this country.

- • We're not anti-anything. The only things we fight are attempts to take away or limit your civil liberties, like your right to practice any religion you want (or none at all)....

- • We're there for you.... Every person in this country should have the same basic rights. And since our founding in 1920, we've been working hard to make sure no one takes them away. The ACLU is our nation's guardian of liberty.... Freedom is why we're here.[1]

Every person in this country should have the same basic rights, declares the ACLU. Human beings called "mental patients" are persons. Hence, they ought to have the same rights as persons not called "mental patients." However, that is not position of the ACLU now, nor has it ever been.

The ACLU's Love Affair with Psychiatric Slavery

During its first quarter of a century, the ACLU took no notice of psychiatric slavery. Once it did, it was love at first sight. Charles L. Markmann, the official historian of the ACLU, proudly relates how, after World War II, the ACLU "began to draft model statutes for the commitment of the insane."[2] The ACLU has never wavered in its support of involuntary mental hospitalization and the insanity defense.[3] Markmann smugly writes:

Having made an initial inroad on *entrenched ignorance* by the overthrow of the California law making narcotics addiction a crime [referring here to the U.S. Supreme Court's *Robinson* decision], the Union, however belatedly, has begun a similar campaign against the parallel callousness that treats the alcoholic as the criminal he is not rather than as *the sick man he is. The Union will attempt to bring the law abreast of medicine and justice.*[4]

Markmann brackets medicine and justice as if their aims were identical. Sadly, they are often mutually antagonistic.[5] In 1971, the ACLU proudly reported: "The ACLU Board of Directors is still polishing its policy on mental commitments...there must be assurance that the individual who is committed will, in fact, be treated adequately."[6] How can such an individual be treated if he has no disease and, in any case, wants to have nothing to do with the psychiatrist who is imprisoning him?[7] While the ACLU is polishing its policy about how best to justify the incarceration of psychiatric slaves, the victims are perishing.[8]

In 1978, my criticisms of the ACLU's support for psychiatric coercion evoked an indignant response from Aryeh Neier, then the executive director of the Union. Instead of considering my suggestion that an organization devoted to civil liberties ought to value individual liberty and personal responsibility more highly than psychiatric imprisonment masquerading as a medical treatment, Neier naively reiterated that the ACLU is seeking "more precise criteria for commitment."[9] The leaders and members of the ACLU regard the coercive psychiatrist as the agent and protector of his coerced victim. They cannot comprehend, much less entertain, the idea of abolishing this pernicious practice in its entirety. Where did the leaders of the ACLU get their ideas about psychiatry? Principally from Karl Menninger, an illustrious psychiatrist, and Ramsey Clark, a prominent lawyer.

Menninger was the acknowledged leader of postwar American psychiatry. A founder of the once-famed Menninger Clinic, he was a president of the American Psychoanalytic Association, a recipient of countless psychiatric honors, and a long-time vice-chairman of the National Committee of the ACLU. His following statements represent the gist of his views:

- All people have mental illness of different degrees at different times, and sometimes some are much worse, or better.

- From the standpoint of the psychiatrist, both homosexuality and prostitution—and add to this the use of prostitutes—constitute evidence of immature sexuality...there is no question in the minds of psychiatrists regarding the abnormality of such behavior.

- The very word *justice* irritates the scientist..... [In a society properly informed by psychiatry,] indeterminate sentences will be taken for granted, and preoccupation with punishment as the penalty of the law would have yielded to a concern for the best measure to insure public safety.

- Some mental patients must be detained for a time even against their wishes.[10]

Clark, a former U.S. attorney general, served for many years as the chairman of the ACLU's National Advisory Council. An avowed socialist, Clark has for many years been one of the most prominent and outspoken opponents of capitalism and the free market. He is a founder of the International Action Center, a group whose nature and goals its website describes as follows: "Information, Activism, and Resistance to U.S. Militarism, War, and Corporate Greed, Linking with Struggles Against Racism and Oppression within the United States."[11] Clark is also a self-appointed expert on the ontology of illness and on mental illness as a cause of crime. He states:

- Most people who commit serious crimes have mental health problems.

- Drug addiction is an illness. Medical science can discover cures and provide care.... Drug users should be placed in a correctional program.... Voluntary participation, *which is the basis for civil commitment*, creates an attitude helpful in achieving a cure.

• Punishment as an end in itself is a crime in our time. The crime of punishment, as Karl Menninger has shown through his works, is suffered by all society.[12]

Fortified by such views, the ACLU has led the legal fight for the therapeutic state: in addition to supporting civil commitment and the insanity defense, it supports medical marijuana, physician-assisted suicide, and every other replacement of the rule of law by the rule of medical discretion.[13]

In his autobiography, Aryeh Neier, now executive director of Rights Watch, an organization supported by George Soros, relates that when he joined the NYCLU in 1963, "I knew little about mental commitment. *The issue was not on the civil liberties agenda.* I had not then read the works of Thomas Szasz, the psychiatrist who had long crusaded against the deprivation of liberty on grounds of mental illness. It came as something of a shock to me to discover that New York State law permitted the involuntary hospitalization of someone for thirty days on the basis of an allegation...that the person needed 'immediate observation, care or treatment for mental illness.'"[14]

Neier identifies himself as a "good guy" simply by saying that his discovery of the mental health laws "came as something of a shock." He does not say what shocked him. That the laws permitted preventive psychiatric imprisonment for thirty days instead of, say, three days? What did Neier and the ACLU do about this shocking situation? They made it more shocking by putting the organization's imprimatur on it. It needs to be added here that evidently it did not occur to Neier that the insanity defense is just as serious an infringement of human rights as is civil commitment: *depriving a person of liberty by depriving him of responsibility on the ground of mental illness and incarcerating him in a "forensic facility" is the mirror image of depriving him of liberty on the same ground and incarcerating him in a "psychiatric center."*[15]

In 1968, Neier formed a special action group in the ACLU, called the Civil Liberties and Mental Illness Litigation Project. This Project was, as I shall show, a mouthpiece of organized psychiatry, devoting its efforts to bolstering the legal foundations of psychiatric coercions and excuses.

Not surprisingly, most psychiatrists love the ACLU, whose official position is that psychiatric deprivations of liberty are instances of *bona fide* medical hospitalization and medical treatment. Psychiatric historians—for the most part apologists for the psychiatric profession—are so offended by my calling involuntary mental hospitalization imprisonment that they misrepresent not only my views but also their place in the chronology of modern psychiatry. This necessitates a brief digression here, to set the record straight.

I began my critique of psychiatric coercions and excuses in the 1950s, when civil libertarians either ignored psychiatric slavery or supported it. Nevertheless, in the vast, multi-author volume *A Century of Psychiatry*, Gerald Grob, an American historian of psychiatric slavery, states: "The best known psychiatric critics included Thomas S. Szasz, R. D. Laing.... A more subtle but equally significant critique came from both the legal profession and civil rights advocates. Both raised fundamental and troublesome questions about involuntary commitment and patients' rights."[16] Grob misleadingly equates my views with Laing's, about which more in a moment. In addition, he implies that it was civil libertarians who "criticized" civil commitment, which is false. The reader would also not learn that I did not *merely criticize* civil commitment and the insanity defense, *I advocated their abolition.*

Kathleen Jones, a prominent British sociologist and historian of psychiatry, explains: "One of the medical conservatives [critical of psychiatry] was Dr. Thomas Szasz, who voiced the alarm of *American psychiatrists in private practice*, insisting that fee-for-service was the only proper basis for *treatment....* When Szasz compared State psychiatry with medieval witch-hunts or the activities of the Spanish Inquisition, many of his readers seem to have *failed to notice that he himself was in private practice—and a Professor of Psychiatry.*"[17] Jones, a devout anticapitalist, seems to believe that no intellectual argument is needed to answer my views. My being paid by persons who seek my services because they find them useful and being a professor of psychiatry are enough for her to invalidate my critique of psychiatric slavery, an institution she perceives as providing "free treatment" for "mental illness" to poor people who crave such treatment but cannot afford to pay for it.

This, I believe, is also the place to correct the systematic misrepresentation of the views of Ronald D. Laing (1927-1989). Psychiatrists and many others who write about psychiatry and bracket my name with Laing's typically state that Laing rejected the concept of mental illness and opposed involuntary mental hospitalization. The opposite is the case. Laing wrote: *"When I certify someone insane, I am not equivocating when I write that he is of unsound mind, may be dangerous to himself and others, and requires care and attention in a mental hospital."*[18]

Laing showed no interest in mental health law and never criticized psychiatry's paradigmatic procedures, civil commitment and the insanity defense. In fact, he explicitly opposed my urging the abolition of psychiatric coercions and excuses. In a review in the *New Statesman* of three of my books—*The Theology of Medicine*, *The Myth of Psychotherapy*, and *Schizophrenia*—Laing rose the defense of psychiatry: "But suppose we *do drop* the medical metaphor. If the rest of us could recognize that what Szasz is propounding are, of course, eternal verities, then psychiatry would disappear, and with it what he calls anti-psychiatry. What exactly would happen next?" He then cites my answer, that "involuntary psychiatry, like involuntary servitude, would be abolished," and comments: "It sounds as though it would all be much the same. It makes one wonder what he is making all the fuss about, whether he is not making a sort of fetish out of the medical model, and a scapegoat out of psychiatry."[19] In short, Laing was accusing me of unfairly criticizing a profession innocent of wrongdoing. In a letter to the *New Statesman*, Anthony Stadlen, an English analyst, corrected Laing:

> Dr. R. D. Laing writes: "But suppose we *do drop* the medical metaphor...." Dr. Laing's new role as the "perfectly decent" defender of psychiatry against Szasz's "insulting and abusive...fuss" calls for comment. Laing is saying, unequivocally, that "it would be all much the same" to him whether involuntary psychiatry be retained or abolished. He is saying "it would be all much the same" whether voluntary interventions, including his own, are intended as medical treatments for illness or as interpersonal counseling, ethical exploration, existential analysis. He implies quite clearly that he is one of "the rest of us" who do use the medical metaphor.[20]

In fact, Laing was not opposed to psychiatric coercion. When it suited his personal needs, he made use of psychiatric coercion even in managing his own family. In 1976, Laing's daughter Fiona, then twenty-four years old, was rejected by her boyfriend. According to John Clay, Laing's biographer:

> She had "cracked up," and had been found weeping outside a church near the family home. [Committed to a local mental hospital, she is given ECT.] He [Adrian Laing] rang his father up and asked him "in despair and anger" what he was going to do about it. Laing reassured him that he would visit Fiona and "do everything in his power" to ensure that she was not given ECT, but when it came to the crunch, as Adrian Laing relates, all he could say was "Well, Ruskin Place [the family home] or Gartnavel [the state mental hospital where Laing received his psychiatric training]—what's the difference?"[21]

Regarding the self-stigmatizing label antipsychiatry, it is worth noting that Lavoisier didn't call himself an "anti-phlogistonian"; he simply maintained that phlogiston was the name of an imaginary substance. I am not an "antisychiatrist"; I simply maintain that mental illness is the name of an imaginary illness and reject psychiatric coercions and excuses.[22]

From Bad to Worse: *The Rights of People with Mental Disabilities*

As subsequent events demonstrated, my criticism of the ACLU's policy regarding psychiatric slavery proved to be much too mild. In 1976, the Union issued a formal *Policy Guide on Civil Commitment*, a document that might as well have been written by the board of directors of the American Psychiatric Association. The *Policy Guide* proclaimed:

> The individual should not be incarcerated prior to a hearing, *except in an emergency*.... During such periods of emergency commitment, no action should be taken on the person which might have a permanent effect, and the use of drugs should be *limited solely to those deemed by the attending physician to be medically essential*.... The individual should be able to refuse any treatment for mental illness, *except such treatment as may be required to prevent the patient from being a danger to others*.[23]

In other words, the psychiatrist ought to have unlimited powers over his patients: all he need do is declare the patient's condition an "emergency" and define his own brutalities as "medically essential." Note the absence in these policy recommendations of any reference to the accused person's mental competence or the credibility of the petitioners seeking his psychiatric imprisonment.

In 1996, the ACLU published a new policy statement regarding involuntary psychiatric interventions, entitled *The Rights of People with Mental Disabilities*.[24] In this document, written by Robert M. Levy and Leonard S. Rubenstein, the ACLU offers a ringing endorsement of every form of inhumanity now practiced by psychiatric slaveholders.

Levy and Rubenstein grace their text with this epigraph by Lionel Trilling: "Some paradox of our nature leads, when once we have made our fellow men the objects of our enlightened interest, to go on to make them objects of our pity, then of our wisdom, ultimately of our coercion."[25] This sounds as if the ACLU were opposed to making "the objects of our enlightened interest" the subjects of our coercions. However, that is precisely the policy it supports. Evidently, the ACLU does not entertain the possibility that former slave Frederick Douglass's wise words might now apply to the psychiatric slave. Douglass pleaded:

Everybody has asked the question…. "What shall we do with the Negro?" I have had but one answer from the beginning. *Do nothing with us! Your doing with us has already played the mischief with us. Do nothing with us!* If the apples will not remain on the tree of their own strength, if they are wormeaten at the core, if they are early ripe and disposed to fall, let them fall! I am not for tying or fastening them on the tree in any way, except by nature's plan, and if they will not stay there, let them fall. And if the Negro cannot stand on his own legs, let him fall also. All I ask is, give him a chance to stand on his own legs! Let him alone![26]

That was the last thing whites wanted to do with the "Negro problem." It is the last thing the ACLU wants to do with the "problem of the mentally ill." To justify the psychiatrist's coercive meddling in the life of the mental patient, the ACLU redefines the meaning of the word "right": "When we use the word *right*, we mean a valid, legally recognized claim of entitlement, encompassing both freedom from government interference or discriminatory treatment and an *entitlement to a benefit or service*."[27] I have shown how this view justifies and leads to the expansion of psychiatric coercions.[28]

Levy and Rubenstein explain: "Commitment infringes the right to liberty…. Yet, unlike criminal defendants, people facing commitment can be preventively detained for behavior that violates no law because the confinement is to an institution, not a prison, and *the purpose is treatment*, not punishment…. At its root *the right to treatment* is an assertion that the government has an obligation not just to protect institutionalized individuals or leave them alone, but to provide services that will improve their lives."[29] This is how ACLU lawyers write.

Levy and Rubenstein recognize that once a person is stigmatized as a mental patient and housed in a mental hospital, he has no rights (unless he is in an exceptionally favorable social position, in which case he is not likely to become a psychiatric victim in the first place). They write: "People who enter a facility on their own rather than through state coercion can, *in theory*, leave as they please, so are not deprived of their liberty by the state."[30] The authors recognize that as soon as a person enters a mental hospital he becomes a psychiatric prisoner. They do not object to this.

"The distinction between a voluntary and involuntary status often exists more in a notation on a chart than in the life of the person whose chart it is."[31] Levy and Rubenstein acknowledge that psychiatrists deprive both voluntary and involuntary mental patients of liberty. They do not object to this either. They have become the mouthpieces of organized psychiatric slavery. Other mendacities abound: "Are communications between patients and clinicians confidential? Yes."[32] No![33]

In *The Rights of People with Mental Disabilities*, Levy and Rubenstein describe, but raise no objections against, one of the most obscene consequences of the pretense that psychiatric coercion is medical treatment: "Almost all states have statutes that require individuals, their families, and their estates to pay the costs of both voluntary and involuntary institutionalization. This practice is often justified under the *legal fiction that even people admitted involuntarily enter into an implied contract with the institution to provide for their care and treatment*. Otherwise, it is asserted, they would be unjustly enriched by having received *services* for which they did not pay."[34]

Levy and Rubenstein say that this policy rests on a legal fiction. "Mental illness" and "dangerousness to self or others because of mental illness" are also legal fictions. Levy and Rubenstein treat such fictions as facts because they want to bring about the results they seemingly justify. They approve of imprisoning innocent persons in psychiatric institutions, even if the "hospitalized" person has no "serious mental disorder": "[M]any minors are admitted against their will, *even when they do not have a serious mental disorder*."[35] Ironically, in the process of justifying psychiatric deprivations of human rights, the authors condemn the institution they set out to defend. They conclude:

> These developments [modern mental health reforms] do not tell the entire story. Many of the people who remain in institutions have been there for two or three decades, sometimes longer. Moreover, while their average daily census has declined, each year state hospitals admit hundreds of thousands of people who remain for weeks, months, and sometimes years. And these figures represent but a small segment of the acute care admissions to all inpatient facilities for psychiatric treatment, *now more than two million people annually.* So in this age of deinstitutionalization, a great many people still find themselves institutionalized.... Recent litigation against psychiatric institutions has brought to light instances where individuals have been kept tied to a bed for days at a time and in seclusion rooms for months on end, where seclusion or restraint is used as a form of staff retaliation, and where people were locked in seclusion to allow others to go to a party.... Restrictions on the use of chemical restraints are difficult to enforce.... The difference between appropriate medication and chemical restraint is often as much a metaphysical as a legal or medical question.[36]

Let me repeat this: "The difference between appropriate medication and chemical restraint is often as much a metaphysical as a...medical question," say Levy and Rubenstein. Whether a particular drug is *appropriate* for what ails a particular patient is a *medical question.* Whether a patient uses a drug *voluntarily,* or whether it is *forcibly introduced into his body by agents of the state against his explicit objection,* is a *political question.*

Nevertheless, the ACLU countenances the farce of defining psychiatric preventive detention as a *medical measure. The Rights of People with Mental Disabilities* ends with a listing of "Resources," ostensibly intended to assist persons with "mental disabilities." In fact, they are intended to enable the relatives of such persons to more easily get rid of their unwanted "loved ones." The "Resources" direct the reader to the U.S. Department of Justice, the ACLU, and NAMI. They do not mention any individual or organization that addresses psychiatric coercion from the point of view of the coerced person.[37] They also misrepresent my views—without actually citing any of my contributions to the subject—by equating them with those of Ronald D. Laing, and dismiss them in a footnote.[38]

Conclusion

A person who looks at the term "American Civil Liberties Union" and is told that it is the name of an organization concerned with protecting the American people's right to free speech would assume that the Union is opposed to incarcerating innocent persons because of what they say. This is far from the case.

- A person has the right to declare that, because of an old contract between God and Moses, a tract of land in the Middle East belongs to the Jewish people; another, to declare that, because of the miracle of transubstantiation, a piece of bread is the body of Jesus; still another, to declare that, because Allah chose Mohammed as his one true prophet, the Sharia is the only legitimate law. One is called a Zionist, the other, a Catholic, the third, a Muslim.

- A person has no right to declare that he "hears voices" that tell him he is Jesus. He is called seriously mentally ill and is locked up in a prison called "hospital."

The ACLU defends the rights of Jews, Catholics, and Muslims to assert their particular interpretations of reality, called "religious beliefs," but does not defend the rights of mental patients to assert their idiosyncratic interpretations of reality, called "delusions." However, assertions categorized as "having delusions," like assertions categorized as "witnessing miracles," are instances of speech acts, hence ought to fall under the protection of the First Amendment. Nevertheless, the ACLU stubbornly maintains: "The only things we fight are attempts by the government to take away or limit individual freedoms. Like your right...to speak out for or against anything you wish."[39]

My criticism of the ACLU's position regarding coerced psychiatric interventions may seem too unkind. I do not think so. Let us recall that, in 1963, when Aryeh Neier joined the ACLU, "The issue [mental commitment] was not on the civil liberties agenda." Neier should have asked himself why it wasn't. He would have found that civil commitment was not on the civil liberties agenda because the ACLU had embraced the psychiatric view that mental hospitalization, like medical hospitalization, is a medical procedure. Let us pause and consider this point carefully.

The official position of the American Psychiatric Association (APA) has always been—as a formal document submitted by the APA to a Senate committee in 1961 stated—that: "We, as doctors, want our psychiatric hospitals and outpatient facilities to be looked upon as treatment centers for sick people in the same sense that general hospitals are so viewed."[40] Psychiatrists maintain that, regardless of whether their interventions are consensual or coerced, they are *bona fide* medical interventions on a par with giving a voluntary medical patient an antibiotic. This is the contention I unqualifiedly reject.

The ACLU, like the APA, maintains that psychiatric interventions forcibly imposed on individuals are, and ought to be treated as if they were, therapeutically and legally identical to medical treatments to which individuals submit voluntarily. In that case, involuntary psychiatric interventions do not belong on the civil liberties agenda, just as dermatological or ophthalmological interventions do not belong on it, because neither impinge on civil liberties and, hence, are not proper subjects for the attentions of this group. Q.E.D.

B. Objectivist Libertarians

8

Ayn Rand

Born in St. Petersburg, Ayn Rand (Alissa [Alice] Rosenbaum, 1905-1982) earned a degree in history at the University of Leningrad. After graduation, she briefly studied at the State Institute of Cinema Arts. In 1926, she emigrated to the United States, became a successful novelist, founded a movement based on her "concept of man," called it a "philosophy," and named it Objectivism. "My philosophy," she stated, "in essence, is the concept of man as a heroic being, with his own happiness as the moral purpose of his life, with productive achievement as his noblest activity, and reason as his only absolute."[1]

Rand was energetic, gifted, and enormously conceited. While she was active, she had a considerable following. Her major novels continue to attract new readers. Unfortunately, she ignored the writings of the classic defenders of liberty, insisted that she was not a libertarian, and regarded herself as a champion of capitalism and freedom *sui generis.* The only person to whom she acknowledged an intellectual debt was Aristotle. A tyrannical woman who tolerated no equals, Rand deified reason but displayed little of it in her personal life. She deserves credit for popularizing free market principles but, in my view, did not add anything of significance to the grand literature of liberty, from Montesquieu to Voltaire, Adam Smith, Acton, Mises, and Hayek.

Revered as the goddess of independence and self-reliance by her (orthodox) followers, she never learned to drive, yet chose to live on a ranch twenty-one miles from her office in Hollywood. She depended on her husband for chauffeuring services, and on her disciple, Nathaniel Branden, for sexual services.

Rand and many of her followers regarded Objectivism as, *inter alia,* a system of psychology, a theory of "mental health," and as a technology for achieving it through "reason." In this chapter, I consider only those aspects of Rand's work that touch on psychiatry and psychotherapy.

Rothbard on Rand

In a hard-hitting critique of the Objectivist movement, published in 1972, Murray Rothbard compared "the Ayn Rand cult" to cults such as Hare Krishna, the Moonies, EST, Scientology, and the Manson Family, each characterized by "the dominance of the guru, or Maximum Leader, who is also the creator and ultimate interpreter of a given creed to which the acolyte must be unswervingly loyal. The major if not the only qualification for membership and advancement in the cult is absolute loyalty to and adoration of the guru, and absolute and unquestioning obedience to his commands."[2] All this certainly fit the Randian movement.

Although Rothbard was antagonistic to Rand's persona and style and his criticism of her movement is harsh, it is supported by the evidence of the autobiographical writings of cult members. Commenting on the split that ensued after Branden freed himself from his role as Rand's sex slave, Rothbard observed: "Rand cultists were required to sign a loyalty oath to Rand; essential to the loyalty oath was a declaration that the signer would henceforth never read any future works of the apostate and arch-heretic Branden. After the split, any Rand cultist seen carrying a book or writing by Branden was promptly excommunicated."

Rand viewed herself, and was seen by her followers, as an all-around genius. In this and many other respects, the Randian and Freudian cults were very similar. Many Randians showed a keen interest in psychoanalysis. Indeed, in the eyes of many of Rand's followers, her lectures on Objectivism became indistinguishable from expositions on psychotherapy and exercises in group therapy:

> But the most important sanction for the enforcement of loyalty and obedience, the most important instrument for psychological control of the members, was *the development and practice of Objectivist Psychotherapy*. In effect, this psychological theory held that since emotion always stems from incorrect ideas, that therefore all neurosis did so as well; and hence, the cure for that neurosis is to discover and purge oneself of those incorrect ideas and values. And since Randian ideas were all correct and all deviation therefore incorrect, Objectivist Psychotherapy consisted of (a) inculcating everyone with Randian theory—except now in a supposedly psycho-therapeutic setting; and (b) searching for the hidden deviation from Randian theory responsible for the neurosis and purging it by correcting the deviation (emphasis added).

The similarities between this process and the teaching of psychoanalysis—especially the "training analysis," required by psychoanalytic institutes—are not coincidental. A quasi-religious indoctrination is,

I have long maintained, intrinsic to "mental health" and "psychotherapy" as fanatical secular religions.[3] I summarized this idea in three ironic aphorisms:

- Orthodox: one who recognizes the divinity of Freud; after proven in battle against dissidents, a candidate for a bishopric in one of the training institutes.[4]

- Training analyst: optician fitting his patient with distorting lenses.[5]

- Psychiatric training: the ritualized indoctrination of the young physician into the theory and practice of psychiatric violence.[6]

"It is clear," Rothbard continued, "that, considering the emotional and psychological power of the psychothcrapeutic experience, the Rand cult had in its hands a powerful weapon for reinforcing and sanctioning the molding of the New Randian Man. Philosophy and psychology, explicit doctrine, social pressure, and therapeutic pressure, all reinforced each other to generate obedient and loyal acolytes of Ayn Rand."

Rothbard's essay is a brilliant piece of writing. It is hard to resist the temptation to quote more of it than is necessary to sketch a picture of Objectivism as psychotherapy. His following observations are particularly important:

> The all-encompassing nature of the Randian line may be illustrated by an incident that occurred to a friend of mine who once asked a leading Randian if he disagreed with the movement's position on any conceivable subject. After several minutes of hard thought, the Randian replied: "Well, I can't quite understand their position on smoking." Astonished that the Rand cult had any position on smoking, my friend pressed on: "They have a position on smoking? What is it?" The Randian replied that smoking, according to the cult, was a moral obligation. In my own experience, a top Randian once asked me rather sharply, "How is it that you don't smoke?" When I replied that I had discovered early that I was allergic to smoke, the Randian was mollified: "Oh, that's OK, then." The official justification for making smoking a moral obligation was a sentence in *Atlas*, where the heroine refers to a lit cigarette as symbolizing a fire in the mind, the fire of creative ideas.... One suspects that the actual reason, as in so many other parts of Randian theory...was that Rand simply liked smoking and had the need to cast about for a philosophical system that would make her personal whims not only moral but also a moral obligation incumbent upon everyone who desires to be rational.

Once again, the similarity to the Freudian cult is eerie: in America, the symbol of a psychoanalyst was a man with a foreign accent on his lips and a cigar in his mouth. Although Rand believed that the core of her philosophy was individualism, her followers tellingly called the group they themselves organized "the Collective." Rothbard commented:

> [T]he top circle was designated in the movement as..."the senior collective."... There was an irony within the irony, since the Randian movement was indeed a "collective."... Strengthening the ties within the senior collective was the fact that each and every one of them was related to each other, all being part of one Canadian Jewish family, relatives of either Nathan or Barbara Branden. There was, for example, Nathan's...first cousin, *Dr. Allan Blumenthal, who assumed the mantle of leading Objectivist Psychotherapist after Branden's expulsion.... Thus, power not liberty or reason, was the central thrust of the Randian movement* (emphasis added).

Rand on Psychiatry

In her voluminous writings, Rand never systematically addressed psychiatry or psychotherapy. From the few references she made to the subject, she emerges as a person who saw through much of the imposture that characterizes the mental health field, but had no particular interest in psychiatric coercions and excuses. Her most extensive comments about psychiatry and psychoanalysis are in letters she wrote to philosopher John Hospers, an early and loyal acolyte. My following remarks are based on Rand's letters to Hospers, in which, for the most part, she repeated his questions verbatim before answering them.

Hospers was obsessed with psychoanalysis, which he conflated and confused with both psychotherapy and psychiatry. In her first letter, dated April 17, 1960, in reply to a liberal-anticapitalist comment by Hospers, Rand wrote: "By now, you probably know the exact nature and reasons of my views on capitalism. So I will not attempt to argue with the allegations that capitalists are vicious, exploiting, and warmongering that you make against it—I will say only that I do not agree with you."[7]

On November 27, 1960, she began her fruitless effort to disillusion Hospers about psychoanalysis: "I take issue with your sentence on purely epistemological grounds: [Quoting from Hospers's letter to her] 'As long as we accept the statement that there *are* causes for human behavior, why need one be so alarmed that Freud has discovered what some of these causes are?'... Freud did not discover any actual *causes* of human behavior...."[8] Hospers believed that behavior has *causes* and that Freud made *discoveries*. His gullibility about psychoanalysis and psychiatry made a convenient foil for Rand's ripostes.

Rand may have had many faults but stupidity was not one of them. She had a healthy skepticism about doctrines based on nothing but authority, her own excepted. She saw clearly the reductionistic fallacy in psychoanalysis and in Hospers' thinking: understanding how a person's body works is not the same as understanding the reasons for his actions: "If I were the first scientist who discovered some of the things that man can do with his vocal chord, this would be valuable, but it would not entitle me to declare what songs all men could sing at a certain time nor why they would want to sing them.... If Freud discovered that men have the capacity to practice repression, this does not entitle him to declare that what they repress is the desire to sleep with their mothers or fathers."[9] Psychiatrists, the public, and the media are still hung up on this simple point: they believe that PET scans of the brain showing larger than average-sized ventricles explain "schizophrenia," that is, why a person *claims* he is Jesus, instead of, say, his next-door neighbor.

"You say, 'I don't see how anything that Freud says conflicts with anything that you want to defend.' John, I cannot believe that you mean that...."[10] Like Freud, Hospers wanted to see man as weak, a rider controlled by his horse, to use one of Freud's famous metaphors. In contrast, Rand, like Acton and Mises, wanted to see man as strong, a moral agent responsible for his actions. "'You say,' wrote Hospers, 'I think your aim is the same as Freud's—to help people behave in a rational manner. You do it by appealing directly to reason, Freud does it by helping people incapable of it become capable of it, and thus living by your philosophy. You should not regard him as an enemy.'"[11]

Hospers was confused. He conflated philosophy with psychotherapy, believed that psychotherapy is medical treatment and mental illness is a real disease, and never asked himself how conversation can cure a real disease. To paraphrase Josh Billings, Hospers knew everything about psychiatry that ain't so. Hospers pleaded with Rand: "You say: 'I can't imagine why your group is so opposed to Freud. How do you suppose that *psychiatry* achieves its good effects on patients?'"[12] Hospers refers to Freud as if he had been a psychiatrist, which he was not; to psychiatry as if it were psychoanalysis, which it is not; and to psychiatry as achieving good effects on patients. One wonders what good effects Hospers had in mind.

Rand's nineteen-page letter to Hospers written on April 29, 1961 is especially informative about both of their views on psychiatry. Hospers, still obsessed with "helping" people who could not afford the expenses of psychoanalysis, queried Rand about "free" psychoanalysis.

Rand correctly replied "You ask whether I would be opposed to the 'unofficial rule' of European psychoanalysts to treat one patient free for every ten paying patients. Yes, indeed, I am most profoundly opposed to it...."[13]

Hospers regarded the fashionable liberal-totalitarian practice of using psychiatric imprisonment, renamed "treatment," for punishing criminals as a boon for the "patient." Rand sharply reprimanded him: "This last point, I believe, is the question you are specifically interested in, when you write: 'I find it difficult to say whether a man who has committed, e.g., armed robbery, deserves one year in jail, five years, ten years, or *psychiatric therapy* to keep him from repeating the offense."[14] Did Hospers ask himself whether, charged with a traffic violation, he would prefer to be punished with psychiatric imprisonment or a fine? Hospers's foolish therapeutic compassion epitomized what Rand most hated. Still, she saw him as a potential candidate for recruitment into the Randian ranks. Her following comments are eloquent testimony to her intelligence and courage to see through the sacred dogmas of law-and-psychiatry:

> What punishment is deserved by the two extremes of the scale is open to disagreement and discussion—but the principle by which a specific argument has to be guided is *retribution*, not *reform*.... The purpose of the law is *not* to prevent a future offense, but to punish the one actually committed. If there were a proved, demonstrated, scientific, objectively certain way of preventing future crimes (which does not exist), *it would not justify the idea that the law should prevent future offenses and let the present one go unpunished*. It would still be necessary to punish the actual crime. Therefore, "psychiatric therapy" does not belong—on principle—among the alternatives that you list. And more: it is an enormously dangerous suggestion.... Since the *prevention* of crime is a *psychological* issue, since it involves a man's *mind* (his premises, values, choices, decisions), it would be monstrously evil to place a man's mind into the power of the law, to let the law prescribe and *force upon him* any course of treatment involving or affecting his mind. If "*the prevention of crime*" were accepted as the province and purpose of the law, it would permit and necessitate the most unspeakable atrocities: not merely psychological "brainwashing," but physical mutilations as well, such as electric shock therapy, prefrontal lobotomies and anything else that neurologists might discover. No moral premise—except total altruistic collectivism—could ever justify that sort of horror...*a penal code has to treat men as adult, responsible human beings*; it can deal only with their actions and with such motives as can be objectively demonstrated (such as intent vs. accident); it cannot assume jurisdiction over men's minds, brains, souls, values and moral premises—it cannot assume the *right* to change these by forcible means.[15]

Rand's comments, with which I agree, would have been even better had she given credit for similar opinions to writers who preceded her, such as G. K. Chesterton and C. S. Lewis. Although Rand clearly perceived that psychiatrists have no valid criteria or methods for making the sorts of claims they make, and that involuntary psychiatric interventions are indistinguishable from punishments, she nevertheless cautiously approved of civil commitment: "If a man is *proved* to be legally irresponsible, that is, insane, it is a different issue: the law then has the right to commit him to an insane asylum—since, being incapable of reasoning, he is unable to claim the rights of a rational man. But even then, the law does not have the arbitrary power to impose treatment on him, particularly not treatment that might result in physical damage or injury. And, *even in cases of insanity, the issue of proving it is enormously complex, controversial and dangerous, since no fully demonstrated, scientific knowledge is yet available on what can be taken as proof.*"[16]

For all this, Rand deserves far more credit than she has received. At the same time, many persons who knew Rand well reported that she was fond of calling people with whom she disagreed "crazy." Justin Raimondo recounts that after listening to a "typical vitriolic Randian barrage" against a friend of his, Rothbard felt that "anyone who is not now or soon will be a one-hundred percent Randian Rationalist is an 'enemy'...as well as crazy."[17] She also "held [at least prior to 1954] that anyone who believed in free will was 'insane'—a favorite charge of hers, as Rothbard puts it."[18]

Finally, we must not overlook that, despite the Tolstoyan proportions of Rand's novels, there is no room in them for children. In what has become a famous review of *Atlas Shrugged* in *National Review*, Whittaker Chambers seized on this element and extrapolated it to a conclusion about Rand that, albeit exaggerated, commands consideration. The following is a brief excerpt:

All Miss Rand's chief heroes are also breathtakingly beautiful.... So much radiant energy might seem to serve an eugenic purpose. For, in this story as in Mark Twain's, "all the knights marry the princess"... Yet from the impromptu and surprisingly gymnastic matings of heroine and three of the heroes, no children—it suddenly strikes you—ever result. The possibility is never entertained. And indeed, the strenuously sterile world of *Atlas Shrugged* is scarcely a place for children. You speculate that, in life, children probably irk the author and may make her uneasy.... Something of this implication is fixed in the book's dictatorial tone, which is much its most striking feature.... [R]esistance to the Message cannot be tolerated because disagreement can never be merely honest, prudent or just humanly fallible. Dissent from revelation so final (because, the author would say, so reasonable) can only be willfully wicked. There are ways of dealing with such wickedness, and, in fact, right reason itself enjoins them. From almost any page of *Atlas Shrugged*, a voice can be heard, from painful necessity, commanding: "To the gas chambers—go!"

This is a bit over the top. Chambers's theatrical flourish does not do justice to Rand's principled rejection of initiating the use of force. Being an authoritarian person is one thing. Initiating violence is quite another. And yet, Chambers detected a deep flaw in Rand's character that was there and was not just maliciously imputed to her.

Conclusion

Not being a student of Rand's writings, I wanted to make certain that I was not missing something she wrote about psychiatry that deserved to be mentioned. On March 24, 2003, I sent an email to Rand scholar Chris Matthew Sciabarra, author of *Ayn Rand: The Russian Radical*, asking for his assistance. [19] The next day I received a very helpful, detailed reply. I reproduce below one of my questions to Sciabarra and his answer:

> Szasz: It is my understanding that Rand used terms such as mentally ill and irrational to criticize/dismiss critics. Has she explicitly rejected the psychiatric incarceration of "insane" persons? My impression is that she sidestepped a confrontation with psychiatry. Because of Rand's voluminous writings, most of which I have not read, I could be very mistaken.

> Sciabarra: Well, aside from the fact that she sometimes psychologized with regard to her critics, she did believe that the nexus of psychiatry and the state was lethal. Unfortunately, she never wrote formally on the subject, but she did mention it in a few lectures (most notably, in remarks when she delivered a lecture called "The Moral Factor").... Finally, in the Question and Answer period following her April 1976 address at the Ford Hall Forum, "The Moral Factor," somebody from the audience asked her about your work. She said she'd not read enough of you "to form a full opinion, but what I have read is very interesting." She had some "serious questions" about your premises, but said you seemed to be an advocate of individual rights and that your work was very "promising." As far as I could tell, this is all that one finds that might be directly relevant to your query. [20]

It is not clear what premise of mine she found faulty. It could not have been my *basic premise* that, in its literal-medical use, the word "disease" refers to pathological alterations in cells, tissues, or organs, rendering the term "mental illness" a figure of speech. The evidence suggests that Rand—like most people then, and now—did not scrutinize the semantic foundations of medical and psychiatric epistemology. In one of her letters to Hospers, she wrote: "*Neurosis is a disease and has to be treated as such: it is the subject matter of a special science* and is not the basic and central concern of philosophy."[21] What kind of disease did Rand think neurosis was? Like most people, Rand embraced psychiatry's prevailing premises and prejudices. Despite her own eccentric lifestyle, she condemned homosexuality, calling it "a manifestation of psychological 'flaws, corruptions, errors, unfortunate premises.'"[22] Ironically, she lived long enough to see the American Psychiatric Association abolish the disease status of homosexuality. Twelve years after her death, even "neurosis"—one of the core concepts of psychoanalysis and pre-drug psychiatry—disappeared.[23] It became "mental disorder," just as Alissa Rosenbaum became Ayn Rand.

Despite her glittering intelligence, Rand's fund of information about the hard sciences and medicine seems to have been very limited. In addition, she was inclined to gather around her "followers," a tendency that, in my opinion, is inimical to what I regard as the true spirit of libertarianism. What is that spirit? Ralph Waldo Emerson (1803-1882) put it perfectly: "I have been writing and speaking what were once called novelties, for twenty-five or thirty years, and have not now one disciple. Why? Not that what I said was not true; not that it has not found intelligent receivers, but because it did not go from any wish in me to bring men to me, but to themselves."[24]

In the end, Rand fell into the classic trap of the materialist-rationalist atheist: she believed in the god of reason and rationality, as well as its flip side, the devil of unreason, mental illness.

9

Nathaniel Branden

Nathaniel Branden, born Nathan Blumenthal in 1930, is best known for his intimate association with Ayn Rand. On his website, he identifies himself as follows: "With a Ph.D. in psychology and a background in philosophy, Nathaniel Branden is a practicing clinician in Los Angeles. He lectures and consults with corporations all over the world, teaching the application of self-esteem principles and technology to the challenges of the modern business organization.... In addition to conducting psychotherapy in person in Los Angeles, Nathaniel Branden also consults worldwide with clients via the telephone."[1]

In 1950, Branden became an acolyte of Objectivist cult leader Ayn Rand, and five years later, her paramour. After being expelled from Rand's cult in 1968, Branden moved to Los Angeles, established himself as a psychologist, stopped calling himself an "objectivist," and started calling himself a libertarian. He is the author of numerous books, among them *The Psychology of Self-Esteem*, *Breaking Free*, and *Judgment Day*.

Branden's views on mental illness and psychotherapy do not deserve serious attention. I present them only because many libertarians regard him as a representative of "libertarian psychology and psychotherapy." They ignore, as does Branden himself, the caveat of the great American philosopher, Charles Sanders Peirce (1839-1914): "Consider what effects, which might conceivably have practical bearings, we conceive the object of our conception to have. Then, our conception of these effects is the whole of our conception of the object."[2] The consequences of the contemporary concept of mental illness are incarcerating innocent persons, excusing persons guilty of crimes, and countless other infringements of individual liberty and personal responsibility. It is disingenuous, if not dishonest, to discuss and defend the concept of mental illness and ignore this essential aspect of it.

The Psychology of Self-Esteem

In 1969, having established himself as a psychotherapist, Branden published *The Psychology of Self-Esteem*, grandiosely subtitled, *A New Concept of Man's Psychological Nature.*[3]

The Psychology of Self-Esteem is an unrelenting celebration of psychological discoveries made by himself and Ayn Rand. Branden ignores or is unaware of the works of moral and political philosophers, psychiatrists, psychologists, psychoanalysts, and their critics. The following excerpts convey the flavor of his writing: "The Objectivist epistemology, metaphysics and ethics are the philosophical frame of reference in which I write as a psychologist...for many years...it was my practice to designate my system as 'Objectivist Psychology'."[4]

To make his system (seem) "scientific," he calls it both "Objectivist" and "Biocentric." The term "Objectivist" suggests that there is something wrong with "subjectivism," even when our subject is the beliefs and behaviors of persons with a *subjective, private sense of self and the world about them*. This is an otiose attitude. As for the term "Biocentric," it reeks of pretentious scientism. Declares Branden: "[P]sychology must be firmly rooted in a biological orientation.... I call my system: *Biocentric Psychology*."[5]

Throughout his writings, Branden displays an exaggerated sense of self-importance and uncritical reverence for Rand as a psychologist. He cites this gem from her opus: "The key to...'human nature'...is the fact that man is a being of *volitional consciousness*."[6] This is nonsense. Volition predicates action, not a mental state. Consciousness is not an action and is not limited to human beings. Many animals may be said to possess consciousness.

Branden devotes an entire chapter to "Mental Health." What is his concept of the mind that may be healthy or diseased? He explains: "'Mind' designates specifically *man's* consciousness...in contradistinction to the forms of consciousness exhibited by lower animals."[7] This is a highly idiosyncratic notion of mind and is not the way the term is used, either in everyday language or in the specialized idioms of psychiatry, psychology, and law. Regarding the health and illness of "man's consciousness," Branden writes:

> One of the prime tasks of the science of psychology is to provide *definitions of mental health and mental illness. Psychological disorders are recognized to be the foremost health problems in the nation.* These disorders far surpass any group of physical diseases (such as heart disease or cancer) with

regard to number of victims, economic costs, and general devastation of lives. *More than half of the hospital beds in this country are occupied by the mentally ill.*[8]

Branden proudly identifies himself with psychiatrists and other mental health professionals: he believes that mental illnesses exist and that, ontologically, they belong in the same class as physical diseases, such as AIDS, diabetes, or cancer. *Comme il faut*, he ignores the coercions and excuses intrinsic to the legal and psychiatric uses of the term "mental illness." The persons who typically deploy the term "mental illness" to coerce and excuse people are judges, legal scholars, and practicing attorneys. Yet Branden does not mention the opinion of a single psychiatrist, psychiatric critic, judge, or legal scholar. He also docs not mention psychiatric drugs, mental hospitals, involuntary mental hospitalization, the insanity defense, suicide, and homosexuality.

Evidently, Branden considers none of these issues important. What he focuses on instead is the "mind," an "entity" whose "condition" Branden claims to have special expertise in diagnosing and treating: "The health of a man's mind must be judged by how well that mind performs its biological function. What is the biological function of the mind? Cognition—evaluation—and the regulation of action.... The concept of mental health pertains...to man's 'psycho-epistemology.'"[9] In a footnote, Branden credits Rand with first using this term and adds: "However, the *concept* of 'psycho-epistemology'...was originated neither by Miss Rand nor by myself, but by Barbara Branden."[10] All ideas worthy of notice by Branden are traced to the minds of members of the Randian cult.

What is psycho-epistemology? *"Psycho-epistemology is the study of the nature of, and the relationship between, the conscious, goal-setting, self-regulatory operations of the mind, and the subconscious, automatic operations."*[11] This sentence appears on page 93. On page 26, Branden writes: "'Mind' designates specifically *man's* consciousness...." Clearly, Branden uses words to impress—himself and others—not to understand or explain.

"Mental health is the unobstructed capacity for reality-bound cognitive functioning.... Mental illness is the sustained impairment of this capacity."[12] This is a restatement of the standard psychiatric formula about "reality testing" and its impairments. Branden does not say who has, or ought to have, the authority to determine what counts as "reality-bound cognitive functioning." Presumably, he considers himself well qualified to make such a determination.

"Mental illness is, fundamentally, psycho-epistemological; a mental disorder is a thinking disorder. This is fairly obvious in cases where the patient's predominant symptoms are hallucinations, delusions...."[13] Branden appears to be unfamiliar with the vast psychiatric literature on schizophrenia, whose popularized version he presents as if it were his own discovery. As usual, he ignores the almost equally vast literature critical of the concept of schizophrenia as a disease. Like Rand, Branden writes as if every repetition of a philosophical or psychiatric commonplace sprang straight out of his own intellectual exertions.

Nonsensical assertions of all kinds flow readily from Branden's pen: *"Social metaphysics is the psychological syndrome that characterizes a person who holds the minds of other men, not objective reality, as his ultimate psycho-epistemological frame of reference."*[14] *Webster* defines metaphysics as "a system of first principles or philosophy underlying a particular study," and syndrome as "a group of symptoms or signs typical of a disease." Metaphysics cannot be a syndrome. But Branden can pretend to be a philosopher and expert on nosology.

When Branden considers sexual relations between men and women, he enthusiastically repeats shopworn stereotypes as if they were basic principles of scientific psychology. For example: "[M]an experiences the essence of his masculinity in the act of romantic dominance; woman experiences the essence of her femininity in the act of romantic surrender... it is he who penetrates and the woman who is penetrated."[15] Whom is he kidding? Did Ayn Rand surrender to him? According to Branden's own account, it was *he* who abjectly submitted, and *she* who triumphantly dominated.

There is much more of this kind of drivel. "Thus, sex is the ultimate form in which man experiences *perceptually* that he is good and that life is good.... Sex is the highest form of *selfishness* in the noblest sense of that word."[16] Branden is not only wrong, he is offensive. How can selfishness be noble? It may be necessary, prudent, wise, and self-protective, but noble? Branden's views on ethics are, to put it mildly, lamentable. "There is," he asserts, "no value-judgment more important to man... than the estimate he passes on himself."[17] This value judgment is more important than the prohibition of murder, assault, and theft?

Does Branden believe in mental illness? He does, and with a vengeance: *"Psychotherapy is the treatment of mental disorders by psychological means....* Effective psychotherapy requires a conscious, rational, scientific code of ethics based on the facts of reality...*it is my conviction that Ayn Rand has provided such a code of ethics in her philosophy of*

Objectivism.... But if sacrifice is a virtue, it is not the neurotic but the rational man who must be 'cured."[18] Can ethics be scientific? Can sacrifice never be a virtue? Only a childless person could entertain such ideas. If parents made no sacrifices for their children, few would survive, much less become competent, self-supporting, adults capable of love.

"*A therapist is a scientist.*"[19] Not true. "Every therapist should acquire skill in the art of question-asking under hypnosis, in hypnotic age-regression, and in other related techniques."[20] Wrong again.[21] I am well aware that academic credentials are not evidence of competence. The incomparable Lord Acton earned no "academic degree in his life, not even a high school diploma."[22] Yet, it is worth noting that when Branden wrote *The Psychology of Self-Esteem*, he did not yet have a doctorate in psychology. In the back of the book, he identified himself as "Executive Director of the Institute of Biocentric Psychology and holding an M.A. degree from NYU."

Breaking Free

Breaking Free, published in 1970, is a thoroughly dreadful book. "I had not foreseen," explains Branden, "that I would write a book that would deal, in this manner, with the psychological *problems of children*; nor a book that would be, in part and by implication, a *primer on child-raising*. But every therapist is and must be a child psychologist to some extent—if only because the child is still there, inside the neurotic adult whom we are treating. *He is there, and he is screaming*. This is the story of what he is screaming about."[23]

Branden presents his views as a series of dialogues. He identifies his interlocutors by their first names. They are "Jack," "Robert," "Leonard" and so forth. He identifies himself as "Branden." This semantic accurately reflects Branden's disdainful, authoritarian attitude toward his clients. The text itself is a mixture of pop psychology and self-praise." [S]ince self-esteem is a basic psychological need, the failure to achieve it leads to disastrous consequences and, in fact, underlies all neurotic disorders."[24] Modestly, Branden adds: "The Discovery of the Method...no doubt that I had discovered a potent tool of therapeutic investigation."[25]

At the end, in the "About the Author" note—written by Branden or with his approval—we are informed: "With the publication of his book *The Psychology of Self-Esteem* in 1969, Nathaniel Branden...launched a psychological revolution. He presented a brilliant new concept of human nature, of mental health and illness...."[26] Branden did no such thing.

He created "The Institute of Biocentric Psychology (Biocentric Psychology is the name Mr. Branden has given to his psychological system)," and named himself its "Executive Director."[27] Branden is a genuine cockalorum.

Branden on Mental Illness

As a rule, we assume that persons are responsible for their actions. *If we want to express the idea that a person is not responsible for his actions, we call him mentally ill.* The term "mental illness" entails nonresponsibility, much as term "married person" entails having a spouse. Similarly, we assume that persons who obey the law are entitled to liberty. However, we make an exception for "crazy people." *If we want to express the idea that a person is not entitled to liberty, we call him mentally ill and add the formula, "and dangerous to himself and others."*[28]

These connotations are intrinsic to the operational meaning of the term "mental illness." This is obvious. I emphasize it again because Branden's entire "biocentric psychology" rests on his staunch commitment to the ideas of mental illness and mental health. In an interview, Branded was asked about my views about mental illness. Branden replied: "Szasz's chief contribution, in my opinion, is to have drawn attention to the appalling victimization of mental patients in our psychiatric hospitals, to have emphasized the evil of confining people to mental hospitals involuntarily, and to have warned of the dangerous political implications of 'community psychiatry.' On this subject, I agree with him completely."[29] Branden then added: "I do not, however, agree with his view that mental illness is a 'myth,' and I discuss my reasons in *The Disowned Self*."[30]

Because Branden is so emphatic in his commitment to a belief in mental illness—and also because many libertarians appear to be comfortable in believing in such an "illness"—I shall briefly restate the basis for my objection to it, from a specifically libertarian point of view. The term "mental illness" refers either to an overt act, or it does not. Kleptomania is an example of the former: it refers to stealing and the subject's claim that he cannot help it. Depression is an example of the latter: it refers to a "mental state," feeling grief or suffering. Many persons diagnosed as depressed say that they are not. This intensifies the psychiatrist's diagnostic ardor: he then insists that the "patient" is not only depressed, he also "denies his illness."

As I showed in chapter 2, the libertarian principles of self-ownership and nonaggression render the social uses of the idea of mental illness moot.

If the term refers to a real crime (not simply lawbreaking, as the law often proscribes the exercises of the basic human rights), then the criminal ought to be punished. And if the term refers to a "mental state," then the person—called "mental patient" by mental health professionals—ought to be left unmolested by agents of the coercive apparatus of the state. Since psychologists and psychiatrists are legally and professionally obligated to deprive "seriously mentally ill" persons of liberty, they cannot be both libertarians and mental health professionals. (I am called a psychiatrist, but am not a psychiatrist. I do not believe in and do not treat mental illness.[31])

"Ideas have consequences," Richard Weaver cautioned.[32] So, too, have the words that express them. Such consequences depend on social context. The term "heretic" is harmless when uttered by a clerical worker in America. It is not harmless when uttered by a Muslim cleric in Saudi Arabia. Similarly, the term mental illness may have no (serious) consequences when pronounced by a layperson. However, it has far-reaching, usually devastating, consequences when pronounced by a psychologist or psychiatrist, especially in a legal setting. Branden makes constant use of the term "mental illness," without repudiating its consequences. His devout belief in mental illness negates his protestations about the importance of individual liberty and personal responsibility.

Everyone is familiar with the many ways people use the term "mentally ill"—or a synonym, such as crazy or insane—to excuse themselves or others of responsibility for their bad behavior. The insanity defense—requiring a "diagnosis" of mental illness by accredited psychiatrists or psychologists—epitomizes the magical-religious role that the idea of mental illness plays in law and everyday life.[33] Furthermore, the number one criterion for qualification for compensation for *medical disability*—not only in the United States but in all "advanced" societies—is being certified as "mentally ill" by a psychiatrist or psychologist.[34] To my knowledge, nowhere in his voluminous writings does Branden recognize, let alone object to, this aspect of the concept of mental illness.

For more than three centuries, the mad doctor, alienist, psychiatrist, and psychologist has clung to the idea of mental illness, like the priest clings to the idea of God. This is not surprising. Clerics are experts on God and the Devil; clinicians are experts on mental health and mental illness. Branden loves to refer to himself as a "clinician."

Judgment Day

Judgment Day is a difficult book to write about, because it is unabashedly and embarrassingly exhibitionistic. Right at the beginning, Branden tells us: "If Mother suffered from an anxiety disorder, then my father was passive-aggressive. I did not feel close to either of them, although at times I felt sorry for what I perceived to be the joylessness of their lives."[35] Pity is the product of disdain and narcissism.

Branden's wife, Barbara, was an elegant and exceptionally beautiful young woman. Ayn Rand, married to Frank O'Connor, was twenty-five years older than Branden. To make themselves comfortable about their sexual liaison, Rand and Branden secured the consent of their respective spouses. This arrangement epitomized their idea of rational living. "That we made love in Ayn and Frank's bedroom," Branden writes, "was sometimes hard to bear. *And yet it remained the symbol of our relationship at its most harmonious.... When she looked at me, it was with the eyes of a priestess contemplating the object of her worship.*"[36]

Branden describes Rand as having a "psychological theory" about everything. Years later, he seems still unaware that Rand was a master self-justifier: whatever she did was "rational." Barbara is unhappy with her husband playing the role of Rand's sexual valet-idol. In Branden's presence, Rand lectures Barbara: "'This does not mean that Nathan does not love you,' Ayn went on, 'just as I love Frank. You must understand that.'... 'Barbara,' I [NB] said softly, 'what's happened between Ayn and me had to happen. It changes nothing about how I feel about you,' I meant it."[37] Barbara remained "nervous."

Branden tell us that, in school, he was a poor student, interested only in psychology: "I did not have Ayn's sense of history or her factual knowledge of the past, and while yesterday's traditions meant very little to her, they meant even less to me. *She* was the only tradition that interested me and it lay in the future, not the past."[38] These two non-scholars, interested only in themselves, were truly meant for each other.

Branden begins to pursue his interest in what he calls "psychology": "The first paper I wrote, chiefly inspired by my efforts to understand Barbara and Frank, was entitled 'The Emotionalist Metaphysics.'"[39] He offered this "analysis" of Barbara's mental state: "A few months after the affair began, Barbara awakened one night, in a state of terror. Concerned that she might be having a heart attack, we summoned Allan Blumenthal [Nathaniel's cousin, a psychiatrist and also a member of the Rand cult].

It was not her heart but her mind and emotions that had been stricken."[40] Branden says Barbara's "mind had been stricken." I disagree. It was Barbara the *person who was "stricken"*; more precisely, Branden and Rand *deliberately hurt her, not physically, but psychologically, by their behavior and words.*

Many years after this episode, Branden's and Barbara's perspectives on it are still astonishingly self-deceptive. Branden writes: "I was familiar with the phenomenon of *anxiety disorders.... No* one proposed *medication* and I was not yet aware of the early *tranquilizers* that existed."[41] In *The Passion of Ayn Rand*, Barbara's account of the same events, she writes: "It was Nathaniel who arrived...[at the correct diagnosis] 'pathological anxiety'... This, as in retrospect I understand what was happening to me, names it precisely: the conflict between 'I must' and 'I can't'—the collision of two absolutes. One absolute was that I *must* accept my husband's love affair with Ayn, that it was right, it was rational—the other was the absolute screaming silently within me that *'I can't.'*"[42] In a footnote, she adds: "According to recent scientific findings, *pathological anxiety* is believed to be *primarily the result of a chemical imbalance in the brain... and is treatable with appropriate medication.*"[43] This is what happens when psychologists—who cannot tell the difference between the pancreas and the parathyroid—play doctor.

Nathaniel and Barbara talk to themselves and each other in psychobabble. She refers to her conflicting desires as "absolutes." She does not say what makes these particular desires "absolutes." Suppose she wanted to eat chocolates all day and remain slim. Would those conflicting cravings constitute "absolutes"? Nathaniel labels Barbara's anxiety "pathological," Barbara labels her own anxiety "pathological," and both attribute it to a "chemical imbalance in the brain." The mind boggles. Intellectual arrogance mixed with medical ignorance, serving the cause of self-deception, seemingly has no limits. If Branden had beaten his wife and broken her jaw, would they still have attributed the pain in her jaw to a chemical imbalance in her brain?

Branden and Rand abused Barbara by rubbing her nose in their sexual intimacies. They then they abused her once again, by classifying her unexpressed anger at them as a form of mental illness. They continued to abuse her, "treating" her for her "mental illness." And they abused her some more by "studying" and writing "papers" about her "pathology." Branden explains: "Eager for an explanation [for Barbara's anger at them], Ayn drew on *my theory of 'emotionalist metaphysics'....* She wrote a psychological paper on this subject.... *I had begun to appreciate how widespread the problem of anxiety was, and I was evolving a theory about it.*"[44] In the face of such conceit and narcissism, what can the critic say?

Looking back at Rand and the Collective, Branden writes: "We were not a cult in the literal, dictionary sense of the word, but certainly there was a cultish aspect to our world (in the same way that one might speak, in the early years of psychoanalysis, of 'the cult of Sigmund Freud'...)."[45] This was indeed true, and not only of "the early years."

Today, psychoanalysis is still a cult or, more precisely, several cults. The Nathaniel Branden Institute was also a cult. All schools of psychotherapy are cults. Branden believes that modern schools of psychotherapy—especially his own—are sciences. His naiveté is intact: "Today, of course, there is much wider appreciation of the way *hypnosis can be helpful in all the healing professions.*"[46]

Soon, Branden becomes a devotee of the fashionable "medical" version of psychiatric quackery: "My own tendency was to think more biologically.... The term *biocentric* (life-centered) had not yet entered my vocabulary."[47] Rand might not have known much about psychiatry, but she could smell fraud. "When I tried to tell her of some new research that suggested that certain kinds of depression had a biological basis, she answered angrily, 'I can tell you what causes depression. I can tell you about rational depression and I can tell you about irrational depression—the second is mostly self-pity—and in neither case does biology enter into it.'"[48]

By the time Branden arrives at the end of his story, he is ready to diagnose Rand as mentally ill as well: "In her grandiosity and suspiciousness, *her behavior bordered at times on paranoia, although that is not a thought I would have permitted myself....* I did not attach significance to the fact that, *since her late twenties, she had been taking amphetamines daily*, on the advice of a physician for weight control."[49] Rand was dependent not only on amphetamines but cigarettes as well. She died of cancer of the lung.

In the end, Branden "betrays" Rand by beginning a secret sexual relationship with Patrecia, a much younger and much better looking woman. He asks Barbara, who is still his wife, whether to tell Ayn. "'No. Not about Patrecia. The idea that she was being rejected for Patrecia would kill her.'... If Ayn is 'insane,' I told myself, I have contributed to it.... By not holding her *to the original agreement of 'one or two years at the most.'* By feeding her grandiosity from the day we met."[50]

Did Branden make an agreement with Rand that he will sexually service her for a limited period only? It was a sordid affair, by any measure. Yet Branden feels "distaste" not about what he did but about writing about it: "I experienced extreme distaste at the thought of writing about my affair with Ayn, although I knew that if I did not communicate the actual nature of our relationship, people would never understand the conflict." What people? What conflict? Who cares? Exhibitionism and grandiosity ooze from every pore of these "rationalist" role models.

Branden divorces Barbara, marries Patrecia, moves to Los Angeles, and becomes a pop psychology guru: "Since coming to California, I had been researching what might be accomplished working with groups."[51] Branden, a latecomer to the California pop psychology scene, makes it seem that he was conducting "research" in it. He launches a "therapeutic-educational program...[whose avowed aim is] to generate *psychological growth*, particularly in the area of self-esteem. The workshop, to be called an 'Intensive,' would be spread over three and a half days...[and would be intended to create] increased self-expression, self-assertiveness, and personal integrity."[52]

An Interview with Branden

Branden has built a veritable business on self-esteem. In her introduction to her 1996 interview with Branden, Karen Reedstrom, editor of the Objectivist publication, *Full Context*, wrote: "The name Nathaniel Branden has become synonymous with 'the psychology of self-esteem,' a field he began pioneering over thirty years ago."[53] The psychology of self-esteem is not a "field," it is a Potemkin's village. In the interest of clarifying how Branden sees himself and his work, I cite some excerpts from Reedstrom's interview with Branden.

KR: What do you think of Barbara's *Passion of Ayn Rand*? In your opinion, was it on the whole an accurate biography?

NB: ...Her treatment of the [my] affair with Ayn and later with Patrecia was off on a number of points and left out a good deal that was important. To some extent, that was understandable. She couldn't know what went on between Rand and me, or Patrecia and me, when we were alone....

KR: Many people have argued that you were less than gentlemanly for detailing so much in *Judgment Day*. Did you have to be so explicit in the sex scenes?...

NB: ...when I wrote the memoir I thought that one of its most interesting features would be a man writing intimately about the experience of being in love. Not many men have done that.... So I was shocked at reactions such as your questions imply—truly shocked. *Judgment Day* is the story of my development told through my relationships with three women, of which the relationship with Ayn Rand is the dramatic centerpiece that integrates the events....

KR: But most people I talked to who read *Judgment Day* thought the sex scenes were unnecessary to the story, that it seemed to them you included them to sell books...aren't the details of a romantic relationship, by its nature, still private, as if they were part of an oral contract?

NB: It's very typical of Objectivists, when they object to something someone does, to have a strong opinion as to motive—in this case, to sell books and make money.... Sex is not a sacrosanct aspect of life separate from all normal activities. Sex is part of life....

KR: ...In January, 1990, *Liberty* magazine published an interview with Barbara in which she described herself as quite "angry" with you. She evidently felt you had portrayed her unfairly. She also felt you had taken inadequate responsibility for some of the actions you took while associated with Rand....

NB: ...I do not know what Barbara thinks was "unfair" in my description of her. She certainly knows that I told the truth about our sexual history. She told someone I had presented her in the book as being, in effect, "the Whore of Babylon."... She told me I was refusing to confront the extent of Ayn's evil and of the harm she had done me and her and everyone else. Edith Efron joined her in this view.... I suggested that she and Barbara would benefit from spending more energy looking inward than always dwelling on how terrible Ayn was....

KR: Rand didn't have any children so she could pursue a career, and a lot of Objectivist couples followed her example. Do you regret not having children now that you so much enjoy your grandchildren [sic]?...

NB: I love children.... And yet, knowing myself, I cannot regret not having children of my own because I am so work-focused....

KR: Would it be better for the Objectivist movement if the full truth about Ayn Rand were known?

NB: Objectivism teaches that nothing good comes from faking reality. It would have been a great gift to her admirers if Ayn Rand had been more honestly self-disclosing....

KR: You've also conveyed that Rand did her admirers a disservice by her own moralistic pronouncements about homosexuality. What's your perspective on this?

NB: ...Ayn had the habit, unfortunately, of flinging moral pronouncements about which she had no knowledge to support her verdicts. So did I, at times. Not a good idea....

KR: Do you consider yourself an Objectivist?

NB: In terms of broad fundamentals, sure.

KR: What are your chief differences with Rand?

NB: The biggest area of difference that I am aware of so far is in psychology. *Most of the time I disagree with Rand's psychological explanations of why people believe what they believe or do what they do....* I think her achievements in epistemology are stupendous....[54]

No one has to have children who does not want to. But a thrice-married childless man's protestation of love of children has a hollow sound. Rand, at least, made no such claim.

Branden as Psychotherapist

It is next to impossible for an "outsider" to know just what goes on between a psychotherapist and his patient. This is true even if the psychotherapist sets forth in writing exactly what he does and does not do with patients. Branden has never explained his method of psychotherapy. All we know with certainty is that he is fond of hypnosis and likes to take a dominant role vis-à-vis his patients. In the absence of information from Branden, we must depend on the accounts of former patients about their therapy with him. Murray Rothbard has given us one such account.

For a disastrous six months in the early 1950s, Rothbard fell under Rand's spell and was, during that period, a patient of Branden's. My following remarks about Branden as therapist are based on Justin Raimondo's biography of Rothbard.[55] It must be noted that when Rothbard related his experiences to Raimondo, he was angry because he felt that Branden had betrayed him. Raimondo writes:

> For a long time, Rothbard had been afflicted by a travel phobia, but he was determined to get over it, and on the recommendation of Rand he signed on with Branden as a patient. The relationship lasted less than six months.... Virtually all of the top Randians in New York City were undergoing the rigors of "Objectivist Psychotherapy" as conducted by Rand's chief disciple, Nathaniel Branden.... This is a recruiting technique common with many cults, which often assume a "therapeutic" guise, and in Rothbard, as we shall see, they had a customer blissfully and somewhat naively unaware of just

what he was getting into.... All of Branden's patients were required to take the lecture course [at the Nathaniel Branden Institute], "Basic Principles of Objectivism," as part of their therapy....[56]

While in treatment with Branden, Rothbard received an invitation to lecture in Georgia [Rothbard lived in New York]. Branden assured him he would be cured of his phobia and ought to accept the invitation. Rothbard did so. But a cure did not materialize on schedule:

> When it became obvious that Rothbard's fear of travel was not about to disappear under the moralistic fulminations of "Objectivist Psychotherapy," a mixture of mind-games and hectoring, as well as endless lectures and classes of "Basic Principles of Objectivism," Branden decided that Rothbard's problem was linked to other issues—for example, Rothbard's "irrational" choice of a mate. For how could Rothbard claim to be rational if he chose a mate whose belief in God violated the Randian principle of the primacy of reason?[57]

Rothbard apologized to the conference organizers: "When I accepted your invitation last winter, I was convinced by the assurances of my therapist, Nathaniel Branden, to whom I had been going in an effort to rid myself of my phobia about traveling that I would definitely be able to attend the conference because I would be cured of the phobia by this fall."[58] Raimondo's comment about this is a bombshell: "It is a quite distraught letter, painful to read, especially when one realizes the extent of the psychological abuse inflicted by Branden on his trusting patient. *The unusual fact that Rothbard was threatened with a lawsuit by his own therapist led to the public revelation of the intimate details of his psychological state*."[59] What was the substance of Branden's threatened lawsuit? In a personal communication, Raimondo explained:

> Branden threatened to sue Rothbard for "stealing" what he believed to be Ayn Rand's "original" contribution to philosophy, the idea that the concept of ethics is derived from the concept of human life as the standard of value. Rothbard was under Branden's "care" at the time.... Branden has set this up [Rothbard's delivering a paper in Georgia] as a kind of test of Rothbard's mental health, and Rothbard was eager to be cured of his phobia about traveling outside of New York City. So Rothbard wrote his paper, and prepared to make the journey, but before he left he showed the paper he had written to Branden—who was outraged. Branden claimed that Rothbard had "stolen" ideas from Ayn Rand, and not given her any credit. An acrimonious dispute ensured, with Branden calling up Rothbard and sending him letters, threatening to sue him—for "stealing" Rand's ideas. Rothbard told him that the ideas expressed in his paper were *not* Rand's "original" contribution, but could be traced back to the Scholastics of the Middle Ages. Branden continued to threaten him with a lawsuit....[60]

If Rothbard's and Raimondo's account is true, Branden's idea of psychotherapy, at least at that time, was to indoctrinate, browbeat, and betray the patient: "For the past six months, Rothbard had confided his secrets, his longings, his anxieties, and poured out his heart secure in the knowledge that Branden's sense of professional ethics and propriety would forbid him to betray such a confidence."[61]

Rothbard found out the hard way that Branden's sense of professional ethics offered no such protection. Raimondo writes: "Branden...had the goods on each and every one of their [Rand's and his] followers... if Rand and Branden decided that this or that Objectivist had deviated from orthodoxy, was unrepentant, and had to be excommunicated from the group, then all this sensitive information was revealed at their subsequent 'trial.' The Grand Inquisitor at these bizarre proceedings was always Nathaniel Branden."[62]

The kind of therapy Rothbard and Raimondo attribute to Branden is, of course, utterly incompatible with the libertarian values of self-ownership, contractual obligations, and personal independence and integrity. Therapists who promise to keep their clients' communications confidential and don't are knaves. Clients who entrust their confidences to such con men of the soul are fools.

Conclusion

In *Judgment Day*, Branden approvingly writes: "One of the most important tenets of Ayn's philosophy, the foundation of her political theory, was that no individual and no group, including the government, has the moral right to *initiate physical force against anyone who has not resorted to its use*."[63] Making a psychiatric diagnosis that justifies involuntary mental hospitalization is an instance of *initiating force against a person who has not resorted to its use*. To be sure, the psychologist (or psychiatrist) is like the judge who issues the order to incarcerate, rather than like the police officer or hospital attendant who escorts the convicted defendant/committed patient to the prison or mental hospital.

If Branden believes that "no individual and no group, including the government, has the moral right to *initiate* physical force against anyone who has not resorted to its use," then he should have denounced all coercive psychiatric and psychological practices. He has not done so in the past and is not doing so now.

I am not the first observer of Branden's career to cast aspersions on his persona and work. Writer Edith Efron characterized him as "a sort of con man." Rothbard dismissed him in even harsher terms: "Old Branden or New Branden, Randian shrink or Biocentric shrink, student or Ph.D., young or old, he's still the same pompous ass, the same strutting poseur and mountebank, the same victim of his own enormously excessive self-esteem."[64]

C. Libertarians

10

Ludwig von Mises

Ludwig Heinrich Edler von Mises (1881-1973) was born in Lemberg, today called Lwow, also spelled Lvov and Lviv, in western Ukraine. Then in the province of Galicia, in Austria-Hungary, Lemberg was a major cultural and commercial center of the empire. Educated at the University of Vienna, Mises became a pupil of Eugen von Böhm-Bawerk and Carl Menger, founders of the Austrian School of Economics. In 2000, the editors of *Liberty* magazine named him the "Libertarian of the Century."[1]

Mises's first book, *The Theory of Money and Credit*, published in 1912, established him as an authority in economics in pre-World War I Europe.[2] However, the end of the war spelled the doom of the gold standard, free markets, and with them, Mises's reputation. Economic statism—variously called étatism, socialism, communism, Marxism, and Keynesianism—became the order of the day. To make matters worse, in 1922, Mises published *Socialism*, predicting correctly but prematurely the breakdown of the communist system.[3] The name of this great, classical liberal became anathema among "progressives" in the new age of Liberalism.

In 1940, Mises emigrated to the United States and, in 1949, published *Human Action*, his *magnum opus*.[4] A pariah among academic economists, Mises, thanks to the efforts of Henry Hazlitt and Lawrence Fertig, "secured a visiting professorship at New York University's Graduate School of Business. His salary was paid by business people and foundations, and he was never to be a regular member of the faculty. The dean, John Sawhill, even lobbied good students not to take Mises's 'right-wing, reactionary' classes."[5]

Undaunted, Mises taught, wrote, and inspired a brilliant and influential group of students to develop and spread the ideas of individual liberty and personal responsibility, based on the right to property and the free market. The Ludwig von Mises Institute, in Auburn, Alabama, is devoted to preserving his memory as the "eminent and noble man" that he was.[6]

Although Mises was considered primarily an economist, he was far more than that: he was a political philosopher and one of modern history's giants in the struggle against the totalitarian state, in all its guises, at war against individual liberty and personal responsibility.

My admiration for Mises's work and persona is unbounded. Hence, it is with some reluctance and regret that I present his comments about psychiatry. His views illustrate that, although Mises thought for himself about economics and politics, he let the prevailing Zeitgeist think for him about psychiatry.

Praxeology and Psychiatry

Mises named his philosophy of economics "praxeology," to denote that its subject matter is human *praxis*, that is, action or performance. In the first edition of *Human Action* (1949), he declared: "No treatment of economic problems proper can avoid starting from acts of choice; economics becomes a part...of a more universal science, *praxeology* [a general theory of human action]."[7]

In contrast to economists who treat their field as if it were a branch of applied mathematics, already in *Socialism* (1922), one of Mises's early writings, he insisted that "It is...illegitimate to regard the 'economic' as a definite sphere of human action which can be sharply delimited from other spheres of action.... The economic principle applies to all human action.... Economics deals with society's fundamental problems; it concerns everyone and belongs to all. It is the main and proper study of every citizen."[8] In *Human Action* (1949/1994), he repeated: "Economics is not about things and tangible material objects; it is about men, their meanings and actions."[9]

According to Mises's definition, the problems that concern economists overlap with those that concern psychiatrists and psychologists and, indeed, ought to concern "every citizen." Yet, Mises himself, and libertarians in general, have not taken seriously enough that this perspective obligates them to subject psychiatric coercions to the same critical scrutiny to which they subject economic and political coercions.

Viewed as the study of human action, economics and psychiatry are fraternal twins: economists are concerned mainly with the material and political consequences of choices and actions; psychiatrists, mainly with their personal and interpersonal consequences. Yet economists and libertarians have shown no interest in psychiatry. Because psychiatry was established as, and has always been, a coercive-statist enterprise—with the *state* mental hospital as its emblematic institution and locus—this is an especially astonishing omission. Of course, neither the economist nor the psychiatrist can avoid trespassing on his sibling's territory. But since the brothers don't speak the same language, each is ignorant about his own flesh and blood.

The profession of psychiatry as a medical specialty rests on the idea of insanity as an illness, epitomized by the individual beset with "irresistible impulses" that transform him from a responsible moral agent into a "mental patient" not responsible for his behavior. That image forms the basis of civil commitment and the insanity defense and affects social policies in modern societies in a myriad ways.[10] Sir Henry Maudsley (1835-1918), the undisputed founder of modern British psychiatry, offered the following account of this basic concept of psychiatry:

> To hold an insane person responsible for not controlling an insane impulse...is in some cases just as false in doctrine and just as cruel in practice as it would be to hold a man convulsed by strychnia responsible for not stopping the convulsions.... [I]t is a fact that in certain mental diseases a morbid impulse may take such *despotic possession of the patient as to drive him, in spite of reason and against his will, to a desperate act of suicide or homicide*; like the demoniac of old into whom the unclean spirit entered, he is possessed by a power which forces him to a deed of which he has the utmost dread and horror.[11]

More than a hundred years later, psychiatrists and psychiatrically enlightened lawyers and politicians hold the same view. Michael S. Moore, professor of law and professor of philosophy at the University of San Diego, writes: "It is not so much that we excuse them [the mentally ill] from a *prima facie* case of responsibility; rather, by being unable to regard them as fully rational beings, we cannot affirm the essential condition to viewing them as moral agents to begin with. In this the mentally ill join (to a decreasing degree) infants, wild beasts, plants, and stones—none of which are responsible because of the absence of any assumption of rationality."[12]

These passages present us with nearly all the moral, medical, linguistic, and legal metaphors and misapprehensions that form the foundations of modern psychiatry. By medicalizing (mis)behavior, psychiatry replaces the otherworldly superstitions of religion with the worldly superstitions of scientism. Without identifying this view with psychiatry, Mises explicitly rejected it: "To punish criminal offenses committed in a state of emotional excitement or intoxication more mildly than other offenses is tantamount to encouraging such excesses.... Man is a being capable of subduing his instincts, emotions, and impulses.... *He is not a puppet of his appetites...he chooses; in short, he acts.... Human action is necessarily always rational.* The term 'rational action' is therefore pleonastic and must be rejected as such."[13]

If all human action is rational, then no action is irrational or, as psychiatrists and their admirers like to put it, "senseless." It is only a short step from Mises's assertion that human action is always rational, to my assertion that mental illness is a myth. Nevertheless, in his many references to insanity, Mises expressed an uncritical acceptance of standard psychiatric mythology.

Human Action *(1949)*

After presenting his case for the moral and economic superiority of cooperation over coercion and anarchy, Mises declared: "Even if we admit that every *sane* adult is endowed with the faculty of realizing the good of social cooperation and of acting accordingly, there still remains the problem of infants, the aged, and the insane. We may agree that *he who acts antisocially should be considered mentally sick and in need of care.*"[14] The same passage appeared five years earlier, in Mises's *Omnipotent Government* (1944), where the last word was "cure," not "care."[15] These are unfortunate statements. The terms "aged" and "insane" do not identify homogeneous groups of individuals, just as the terms "child," "adult," and "sane" do not do so either.

Mises alternately scoffed at psychiatry and uncritically accepted its prejudices. For example:

- "No better is the propensity, very popular nowadays to brand supporters of other ideologies as lunatics. Psychiatrists are vague in drawing a line between sanity and insanity."[16]

- "[I]t is clear that if the mere fact that a man shares erroneous views and acts according to his errors qualifies him as mentally disabled, it would be very hard to discover an individual to which the epithet sane or normal could be attributed.... If to err were the characteristic feature of mental disability, then everybody should be called mentally disabled."[17]

- *"It would be preposterous for laymen to interfere with this fundamental issue of psychiatry."*[18]

On the contrary. The issue here is not merely where to draw the line between sanity and insanity as abstract concepts. The issue is to decide whether an individual innocent of lawbreaking ought to be deprived of liberty, a matter *that rightly belongs to ethics and politics, not psychiatry qua medicine or treatment.* Accordingly, *it is imperative that everyone be concerned with this fundamental issue.* Mises failed to draw the logical conclusion inherent in his own view of human action, namely, that having a delusion ought to be regarded as a fundamental human right, lest all disagreements with authority be potentially disqualified as mental illnesses. We have seen this happening all over the world, notably in the Soviet Union, and see it happening now in Communist China.

Mises was a clear and courageous thinker, except when it came to psychiatry. Then he, too, suspended critical judgment and recoiled from offending this secular religion. For example, he wrote: "If a statement were not exposed as logically erroneous, psychopathology would not be in a position to qualify the state of mind from which it stems as pathological. If a man imagines himself to be the king of Siam, the first thing which the psychiatrist has to establish is whether or not he really is what he believes himself to be. *Only if the question is answered in the negative can the man be considered insane.*"[19] This is embarrassing. Neither "logical errors" nor lies are *symptoms of disease.* Mises knew that persons diagnosed insane are incarcerated in mental hospitals, but remained silent on the subject.

There are many reasons why a man who is not rich might say that he is, and many reasons why a man who is not the king of Siam might say that he is: he may be acting, or lying, or malingering, or protesting his insignificance—his false self-identification a metaphor. Mises would not have suggested that a man is insane because he says that, when he dies, he will go to heaven and be reunited with his dead wife. There is no more empirical or logical ground for suggesting that the would-be King of Siam is insane. (To be sure, there are cultural and social grounds for such a view.)

Liberalism *(1927)*

Written in German, *Liberalism* appeared more than twenty years before *Human Action.* It abounds in psychiatric indiscretions. In the Introduction, Mises declared: "This opposition [to liberalism, a term Mises uses in its nineteenth-century sense], does not stem from the [sic] reason, but *from a pathological mental attitude—from resentment and from a neurasthenic condition that one might call a Fourier complex, after the French socialist of that name*."[20] In the jargon of Freudian psychobabble, Mises continued:

> The *Fourier complex* is much harder to combat. What is involved in this case is a serious disease of the nervous system, a neurosis, which is more properly the concern of the psychologist than of the legislator.... Unfortunately, medical men have hitherto scarcely concerned themselves with the problem presented by the Fourier complex. Indeed, they have hardly been noticed even by *Freud, the great master of psychology,* or by his followers in their theory of neurosis, though it is to psychoanalysis that we are indebted for having opened up the path that alone leads to a coherent and systematic understanding of *mental disorders of this kind.... Only the theory of neurosis can explain the success enjoyed by Fourierism, the mad product of a seriously deranged brain.* This is not the place to adduce evidence of *Fourier's psychosis* by quoting passages from his writings.[21]

No comment is necessary. Happily, Mises's views about drugs, drug addiction, and drug controls remained largely, though not wholly, unaffected by psychiatric bigotry. He declared:

> In the United States, the manufacture and sale of alcoholic beverages are prohibited.... It is universally deemed one of the tasks of legislation and government to protect the individual from himself.... No words need to be wasted over the fact that all these narcotics are harmful...a utilitarian must therefore consider them as vices. But this is far from demonstrating that the authorities must interpose to suppress these vices by commercial prohibitions, nor is the government really capable of suppressing them.... Why should not what is valid for these poisons be valid also for nicotine, caffeine, and the like? Why should not the state generally prescribe which foods may be indulged in and which must be avoided because they are injurious?...[22]

This fine statement is marred by the aside, "No words need to be wasted over the fact that all these narcotics are harmful." Unless we qualify which drugs, in what doses, for whom, under what circumstances, this statement is simply not true. At the same time, Mises correctly located the source of the problem in widespread infantilism and lack of self-discipline: "The propensity of our contemporaries to demand authoritarian prohibition as soon as something does not please them, and their readiness to submit to such prohibitions even when what is prohibited is quite agreeable to them, shows how deeply ingrained the spirit of servility still remains within them. It will require many long years of self-education until the subject can turn himself into the citizen."[23]

In *Human Action*, Mises reprinted the passage about drugs, omitting the reference to Prohibition and adding some powerful lines:

Opium and morphine are certainly dangerous, habit-forming drugs. But once the principle is admitted that it is the duty of government to protect the individual against his own foolishness, no serious objections can be advanced against further encroachments.... [W]hy limit the government's benevolent providence to the protection of the individual's body only?... The mischief done by bad ideologies, surely, is much more pernicious, both for the individual and for the whole society, than that done by narcotic drugs.... These fears are not merely imaginary specters terrifying secluded doctrinaires. It is a fact that no paternal government, whether ancient or modern, ever shrank from regimenting its subjects' minds, beliefs, and opinions. *If one abolishes man's freedom to determine his own consumption, one takes all freedom away.*"[24]

In my book, *Our Right to Drugs*, I carried Mises's final remark to its logical and practical conclusion and showed that the right to ingest anything we please—and poison and kill ourselves, if we so choose—is more fundamental than many other so-called basic human rights.[25]

At the end of *Liberalism*, Mises disappoints: "The League of Nations may continue to combat contagious disease, the drug traffic, and prostitution."[26] And: "[The goal] at which all men aim, is the best possible satisfaction of human wants: it is prosperity and abundance.... To diminish suffering, to increase happiness: that is its [Liberalism's] aim."[27] This view resonates with Bentham too closely for comfort. What Mises says here sounds more like socialist Utilitarianism than laissez-faire Liberalism.

Conclusion

Mises, like Hayek, opposed the pretensions of social science theorizing imitating the physical sciences.[28] But unlike Hayek, Mises was eager to categorize the study of human behavior as a science. In *The Ultimate Foundations of Economic Science* (1962), he wrote: "In dealing with the epistemology of the sciences of human action, one must not take one's cue from geometry, mechanics, or any other science."[29] And again: "An honest man, perfectly familiar with all the achievements of contemporary natural science, would have to admit freely and unreservedly that the natural sciences *do not know what the mind is and how it works* and that their methods of research are not fit to deal with the problems dealt with by the sciences of human action."[30] If the natural sciences—of which neurology and biological psychiatry are branches—do not know what the mind is and how it works, how can they know what a disease of the mind is?

Mises was a great man, not only because he was a great economist but because he recognized that the twentieth century's great collectivist movements of "liberation," National Socialism (Nazism) and International Socialism (Communism), were simply new versions of slavery, and fought tirelessly, and against great odds, against them. He kept his eyes on the right ball: "In the sixteenth and seventeenth centuries religion was the main issue in European political controversies. In the eighteenth and nineteenth centuries in Europe as well as in America the paramount question was representative government versus royal absolutism. Today it is the market economy versus socialism."[31] I agree and add: Today it is also freedom from psychiatric categorization versus the tyranny of the therapeutic state or, more simply, the separation of psychiatry and the state.

11

Friedrich von Hayek

Friedrich August von Hayek (1899-1992) is widely acknowledged as the greatest twentieth-century philosopher of liberty. Hayek called himself a classical liberal, but it is fair to regard him as a libertarian.

Born to a distinguished family of Viennese intellectuals, Hayek attended the University of Vienna, earning doctorates in law and economics in 1921 and 1923. In 1931, he moved to England and spent the war years as a professor of economics at the London School of Economics. In 1950, he joined the Committee on Social Thought at the University of Chicago, and in 1974 was awarded the Nobel Memorial Prize in Economic Science.

The Rule of Law and its Implication for Psychiatry

Hayek was strongly influenced by the work of the great English legal philosopher Albert Venn Dicey (1835-1922). Dicey viewed the constitutional state—what the Germans call *Rechtsstaat*, *Recht* meaning both "right" and "law"—as an organ of coercion with its power limited by law. The rule of law requires that all government action be authorized by law, which binds everyone equally. In this conception, the rule of law is to the political philosophy of individual liberty as our skeleton is to our body. Weakening or removing the former enfeebles and destroys the latter. One of the most insidious and effective ways to accomplish this was, already in Dicey's day, through medicine. In 1905, he warned: "The collectivist never holds a stronger position than when he advocates the enforcement of the best ascertained laws of health."[1] In 1914, Dicey added: "The Mental Deficiency Act is the first step along a path on which no sane man can decline to enter, but which, if too far pursued, will bring statesmen across difficulties hard to meet without considerable interference with individual liberty."[2] Dicey foresaw the day when the quest for mental health would become the number one enemy of individual liberty.

The rule of law was central to Hayek's thought and work on the "constitution of liberty." He wrote: "Under the rule of law, government can infringe a person's protected private sphere *only as punishment for breaking an announced general rule.*"[3] Note that this formulation negates the legitimacy of psychiatric coercions and excuses: abolishing all non-punitive sanctions—epitomized by mental health laws—would liquidate all non-consensual psychiatric relations and thus *destroy psychiatry as we know it.*

Libertarians, as well as other admirers of Hayek's writings, have completely ignored this straightforward implication of taking the rule of law seriously. Year after year, many more Americans are deprived of liberty on therapeutic than on punitive grounds. To the 2 million persons per annum deprived of liberty by mental health laws we must add another 2 million derived of liberty by drug laws. Such persons are typically viewed as mentally ill, suffering from "drug addiction" or "substance abuse," and many are sentenced to "treatment" by "drug courts," evidence of the "therapeutic" ideology animating their punishment.[4] Nevertheless, Hayek shared Mises's blind spot about psychiatry.[5]

Hayek recognized that not everyone loves liberty, that some people prefer to be cared for by others, and that such persons pose a problem for the free society. "It is very probable," he wrote, "that there are people who do not value the liberty with which we are concerned, who cannot see that they derive great benefit from it, and who will be ready to give it up to gain other advantages; it may even be true that the necessity to act according to one's own plans and decisions may be felt by them to be more of a burden than an advantage."[6]

Many persons called "mental patients" rank liberty and responsibility low on their scale of values. How should the philosopher of freedom—or a system of laws committed to protecting individual liberty—treat individuals who, instead of wanting to be free, want to be enslaved? Who, instead of wanting to be adults, want to be children or child-like? Both Mises and Hayek treat persons whom psychiatrists label as "insane" as if they were, in fact, unfit for liberty because, like infants and imbeciles, they lack responsibility. In chapter 5 I showed that this view is erroneous.

Hayek and the Myth of Mental Illness

It is difficult for an individual to free himself of *all* socially correct misconceptions. Hayek seems not to have questioned the mythology of psychiatry. In his *magnum opus, The Constitution of Liberty*, he stated:

The complementarity of liberty and responsibility means that the argument for liberty can apply only to those who can be held responsible. It cannot apply to *infants, idiots, or the insane*. It presupposes that a person is capable of learning from experience and of guiding his actions by knowledge thus acquired; it is invalid for those who have not yet learned enough or are incapable of learning. A person *whose actions are fully determined* by the same unchangeable impulses uncontrolled by knowledge of the consequences or a genuine split personality, a *schizophrenic*, could in this sense not be held responsible, because his knowledge that he will be held responsible could not alter his actions. The same would apply to persons suffering from *really uncontrollable urges, kleptomaniacs and dipsomaniacs*, whom experience has proved not to be responsive to normal motives.[7]

Sometimes, Hayek went out of his way to make unnecessary and inaccurate comments about madmen, such as: "We take it for granted that other men treat various things as alike or unlike just as we do...(though not always—e.g., not if they are colorblind or mad)."[8]

Hayek's biographer, Alan Ebenstein reports that "when he was thirteen or fourteen, he asked all the priests he knew to explain what they 'meant by the word *God*. None of them could. That was the end of it for me.'"[9] Unfortunately, Hayek failed to entertain the same sort of skepticism toward the idea of insanity. On the contrary, his belief in psychiatric fictions has an uncomfortable resemblance to the beliefs of pious persons in religious fictions. For example, he believed in the real existence of "uncontrollable urges" and that the habits of stealing and excessive drinking are real diseases, "kleptomania" and "dipsomania."

Because Hayek is an exceptionally important person in the philosophy of libertarianism, and because the notion of "irresistible impulses"— Hayek calls them "really uncontrollable urges"—is an exceptionally important idea in the philosophy of psychiatry, I shall briefly digress to say a word about this oxymoron.

A human being is both a person and a body, agent and object. When a surgeon requests a patient to consent to an operation, he relates to the patient as a person; when he removes the anesthetized patient's appendix, he relates to the patient's body as an object.

Also, it is possible to relate to another person *as if* he were solely an object—for example, a slave—and then treat him as a commodity or thing. The persecutions-protections of certain classes of people are often rationalized by objectifying their members as non-agents, unfit for, and undeserving of, liberty, and perhaps requiring care as property. However, *we cannot, in good faith, relate to ourselves* as if we were non-agents. It is a performative self-contradiction to say to oneself, "I have kleptomania,

I cannot control my inclination to steal." Once a person recognizes that he has a propensity to steal, it becomes his responsibility to control his criminal and immoral behavior, that is, stop stealing or suffer the consequences. In other words, once a person knows he "has kleptomania," his situation becomes indistinguishable from that of a person who, say, knows he has epilepsy and wants to drive. Such a person is not responsible for having the disease "epilepsy," but—assuming the seizures are controllable with drugs—he is responsible for having seizures; and he is responsible for controlling his seizures if he wants to avail himself of the privilege of driving.

Perhaps Hayek's most serious mistake about mental illness was to accept the doctrinal claim that persons diagnosed as insane by psychiatrists *ipso facto* resemble infants and idiots so closely that they are not responsible for their behavior and hence neither need nor are entitled to liberty.

Psychiatry's assault on the philosophy of liberty has always focused on the claim that insanity annuls personal responsibility. For centuries, alienists, mad-doctors, and psychiatrists have insisted that, like infants and imbeciles, insane persons are not responsible for their behavior. In the modern world, especially after World War II, professionals and laymen, liberals, conservatives, and even many libertarians have embraced that view as empirically valid. It is not.

I reject the proposition that "insanity" is an objectively identifiable condition, like infancy. I regard the concept of mental illness (and its synonyms) as a strategy, a ploy that may be used by family members against other, unwanted family members; by the state against deviant persons; and by individuals for their own benefit (for example, to qualify for disability benefits as mental patients).[10]

The language of psychiatry serves the purpose, *inter alia*, of ensuring that individuals diagnosed as mentally ill appear to conform to the stereotypes of madness—that they be perceived as not the agents of their own (illegal or immoral) actions and therefore not responsible for the legal consequences of their (illegal or immoral) actions.[11] Hayek adopted this language when he spoke of "schizophrenics...whose actions are fully determined." There are no objective tests to determine who is and who is not "schizophrenic," whose actions are or are not "fully determined," who "has" or does "not have" responsibility. *Responsibility is an attribution, not an attribute.* Hayek rightly insists that liberty under law requires the *impartial application of rules* applicable equally to all. Psychiatrists do not do this. Indeed, because their rules lack objective criteria, they could not possibly do this.

When Hayek refers to a hypothetical "schizophrenic" as a person whose actions are not altered by his knowledge that he will be held responsible for them, he is again mistaken. The conduct of such a person is plainly susceptible to influence, to rewards and punishments. Ironically, Hayek's characterization of an individual whose "knowledge that he will be held responsible could not alter his actions" fits the person with deeply held religious beliefs more than it fits the person who likes to drink too much. In both cases, the subject makes choices that accord with his desires and values, at least at the time of his acting.

Hayek's reasoning about schizophrenics also contradicts one of his important principles, namely, that "in public life freedom requires that we be regarded *as types, not as unique individuals,* and treated *on the presumption that normal motives and deterrents will be effective, whether this be true in the particular instance or not.*"[12] When Hayek speaks of "types," he clearly means categories identified by objective criteria (such as "persons accused of crimes" or "persons convicted of crimes"), not categories identified by subjective judgments (such as "un-American persons" or "schizophrenic persons"). Hayek's further specification, that we ought to treat everyone by *presuming* that his behavior is governed by "normal motives...*whether this be true in the particular instance or not,*" requires him to view and treat the innocent as innocent, and the guilty as guilty, regardless of whether they suffer from the real disease of anemia or the fictitious disease of schizophrenia. *According to Hayek's own criteria, both civil commitment and the insanity defense violate the rule of law and are incompatible with the basic legal and philosophical principles that undergird the free society.*

Hayek's insistence that, in a free society, laws must promulgate abstract, general rules is well-founded. This principle is, all by itself, sufficient ground for invalidating the justification for any and all psychiatric coercions and excuses. In a passage that could have been written specifically to refute so-called psychiatric abuses, Hayek wrote: "Because the rule is laid down in ignorance of the particular case, and no man's will decides the coercion used to enforce it, the law is not arbitrary. *This, however, is true only if by 'law' we mean the general rules that apply equally to everybody....* As a true law should not name any particulars, so it should especially not single out any specific persons or groups of persons."[13]

Mental health laws mandating psychiatric coercions prescribe exactly what Hayek says genuine laws ought not to do: they single out "mentally ill" persons and regulate their behavior by special criteria used solely for regulating the behavior of wards of the state—"infants, idiots, and the insane." The criteria of innocence and guilt, used for judging and regulating the behavior of "normal" persons, do not apply to these persons, viewed as human beings but not moral agents.

Hayek on Medicine and Psychiatry

Although Hayek was a learned man, he was, like many scholars of the humane sciences (*Geisteswissenschaften*), remarkably ignorant and misinformed about matters of health, disease, and treatment.

This ignorance, especially with respect to mental illness, was not due to lack of opportunity to learn. Hayek was born in Vienna, in 1899, the year before Freud published *The Interpretation of Dreams*. By the time Hayek entered the Gymnasium, Freud was a famous figure in his hometown and throughout the Western world. So also was Karl Kraus—who was even more popular in Vienna than Freud—among whose pet enemies were psychiatry and psychoanalysis.[14] Alan Ebenstein, Hayek's biographer, tells us that, "While finishing his law degree, Hayek formed a discussion group—the *Geistkreis*."[15] (The German *Geist* stands for both "mind" and "spirit." *Kreis* means "circle" or "group.") Several members of this group later became well-known professionals, mainly economists, for example, Gottffied Haberler, Fritz Machlup, and Oskar Morgenstern. The psychoanalyst Robert Waelder was also a member of the *Kreis*.

From Ebenstein we also learn that "Hayek began to suffer from truly significant depression from about the time of his 1961 visit to Charlottesville, Virginia, which was later diagnosed as in part the reaction to a mild heart attack that was not discovered at that time." Chronically depressed, Hayek's condition worsened in 1969, "when he had another, somewhat more significant, heart attack (also not discovered at that time)."[16]

During most of these years Hayek was at the University of Chicago. The university was, and is, the home of one of the most famous medical centers in the country. The city of Chicago was, and is, the home of other outstanding medical schools and hospitals. Hayek's son, Larry, was a physician. How could Hayek, in 1961 at the age of sixty-two, have two undiagnosed heart attacks? Did he go to doctors to find out what ailed him? Did he avoid doctors? Ebenstein does not say. He adds, however:

> After 1985, significant depression, as well as old age and ill health, struck him.... He attributed some of these problems [depression] to misdiagnosis. He said in a 1985 interview that "there was a period when I was in a very bad state of health. For two or three years I was suffering from what the doctors

called depression. I always said that is nonsense; I am depressed because I can't work, not the other way round. Now there is a modern technique of electrocardiography that discovered that apparently I have had two heart attacks, and the second one knocked me out for three years, and it has only been discovered in retrospect."[17]

Ebenstein relates this without comment, which suggests that he, too, lacks even an elementary familiarity with medicine. Electrocardiography—which, in 1985, Hayek characterized as a "modern technique"—was developed in 1893 by the Dutch physician Willem Einthoven. In the same year, he proposed the terms "electrocardiogram" and "electrocardiography." By the 1930s, electrocardiography was a routine medical procedure. Calling it, in 1985, a "modern technique," as Hayek did, is like calling telephony a modern technique.

The oddity of the alleged misdiagnoses of Hayek's illnesses does not end there. Hayek was a heavy smoker. The causal connection between smoking and coronary heart disease was an established medical fact by the early decades of the last century. After World War II, the correlation was common knowledge, on a par with the knowledge that eating too much causes obesity. This makes it even more odd that Hayek, with his office a few hundred yards from one of the most famous medical centers in the word, was not medically investigated—that he did not seek to be medically investigated—for atherosclerosis and coronary artery disease. In the same interview, Hayek was asked: "Why do you use snuff?" He replied:

Well, I was stopped from smoking by the doctor and was miserable for a long time. I was a heavy pipe smoker. I took some snuff and found the longing at once stopped. So I started taking it up and I've become completely hooked. It is as much a habit-forming thing, and you get all the nicotine you want; but the worst thing about smoking, of course, is the tar, which you don't get. So I get my pleasure without the real danger.[18]

This statement implies that Hayek was aware of the deleterious effects of smoking. But, amazingly, even after learning about this risk, he managed to know "what ain't so."[19] Smoking damages many organs, the lungs mainly by the inhalation of particulate matter, the heart and circulatory system mainly by the chemical action of nicotine. Receiving nicotine through the lining of the nose, as snuff, or the lining of the oral cavity, as chewing tobacco, is just as harmful for the heart as is inhaling it through the lungs by smoking cigarettes.

Hayek's gullible attitude toward medicine contrasts sharply with his skeptical attitude toward religion, mentioned earlier. His incuriosity—indeed, his actively not wanting to know too much about medicine—may explain his ignoring psychiatry as the single most important weapon in the modern state's war against individual liberty and personal responsibility. If Hayek could be as selectively unintelligent about his own medical condition as in fact he was, we could not expect him to have been more knowledgeable about the doings of the doctors called "psychiatrists." Hayek's own contributions to psychology support these conjectures.

Hayek and Psychology

It is impossible to appreciate the complexity of Hayek's work, and persona, without carefully studying his book, *The Sensory Order: An Inquiry Into the Foundations of Theoretical Psychology*.[20] Hayek deemed this to be one of his important works. I regard it as a monumental mistake: its thesis is inconsistent with his perceptive and courageous denunciation of scientism in the social "sciences," and his monumental oeuvre on political philosophy.

The Sensory Order is presented in the style of the logical positivists, as a series of propositions, beginning with 1.1 and ending with 8.98. The first section of the first chapter is headed: "What is Mind?" Hayek does not answer the question. He talks around it and propounds generalities that are either self-evident or meaningless. Throughout, Hayek's language is virtually undecipherable. An impenetrable turgidity permeates the entire text. The following are some of his clearer statements:

> 1.13.... The task of the physical sciences is to replace that classification of events which our senses perform but which proves inadequate to describe the regularities in these terms, by a classification which will put us in a better position to do so. The task of theoretical psychology is the converse one of explaining why these events, which on the basis of their relations to each other can be arranged in a certain (physical) order, manifest a different order in their effect on our senses.... 2.50. This central contention may also be expressed more briefly by saying that we do not first have sensations which are then preserved by memory, but it is as a result of physiological memory that the physiological impulses are converted into sensations.[21]

Paradoxically, Hayek ends *The Sensory Order* on a note that contradicts the whole thrust of the book: "8.98. Our conclusion, therefore, must be that *to us* mind must remain forever a realm of its own which we can know only through directly experiencing it, but which we shall never be able fully to 'reduce' to something else."[22]

Ebenstein states that Hayek "considered his work in psychology to be among the most important of his career." In 1978, Hayek told James Buchanan:

> I think the thing which is really important about it [*The Sensory Order*], and which I could not do when I first conceived the idea, is to formulate the problem I try to answer rather than the answer I want to get. And that problem is, What *determines* the difference between the different sensory qualities? The attempt was to *reduce it to a system of causal connections*, or associations, you might say, in which the quality of a particular sensation—the attribute of blue, or whatever it is—is really its position in a *system of potential connections leading up to actions. You could, in theory, reproduce a sort of map of how one stimulus evokes other stimuli and then further stimuli, which can, in principle, reproduce all the mental processes.*[23]

There were, it seems, two Hayeks. One thought and wrote about persons and groups and states, decisions and actions, slavery and freedom. The other thought and wrote about sensations and causal connections, maps of stimuli and mental processes. Hayek could have saved himself a lot of trouble had he been familiar with an important book by a former member of the University of Chicago faculty. In *Mind, Self & Society*, published in 1934, George Herbert Mead went a long way toward unraveling the problem Hayek set himself.[24] As it happened, Hayek continued to cling to the conventional notion of mind as a private, inner "realm," a conception that leads easily to the view that the mind, like the body, may become diseased.

Regarding Mach's *Analysis of Sensations*, Hayek stated: "My conclusion at an early stage was that *mental events are a particular order of physical events* within a subsystem of the physical world that relates the larger subsystem of the world that we call an organism (and of which they are a part) with the whole system so as to enable that organism to survive."[25] I am afraid this is gibberish, even if it comes from the pen of so great a man as Hayek. Ebenstein's comment: "His work here was also in the tradition of Kant..."[26] Not so.

Instead of critically reflecting on Hayek's work on psychology, Ebenstein is satisfied with situating it in the milieu of the Vienna Circle, logical positivism, and the work of Ernst Mach. Limiting himself to exposition, Ebenstein creates the impression that, somehow, whatever Hayek said and wrote made good sense and was scientifically valid. In *The Sensory Order*, this is emphatically not the case. Ebenstein's biography is unsatisfactory in every way but one: it provides a good deal of raw, useful information.

I might add here that, once upon a time, when I was young, I studied physics and read Mach and the logical positivists. In the late 1950s, when Dover Publications decided to reissue Mach's classic, the publisher invited me to write a new introduction for it, which I did. Its gist was that *The Analysis of Sensations*—an exposition of late nineteenth-century psychophysical parallelism—is largely of historical interest.[27] A brief excerpt from Mach's essay shows that Hayek's *The Sensory Order* is, in effect, a restatement of it. "A color is a physical object as soon as we consider its dependence, for instance, upon its luminous source, upon other colors, upon temperatures, upon spaces, and so forth. When we consider, however, its dependence upon the retina...it is a psychological object, a sensation."[28]

My work on pain in the 1950s was largely inspired by the challenge of unraveling the so-called mind-body problem. In nineteenth-century psychology—then a new "science" pioneered in Germany by Gustav Theodor Fechner (1801-1887) and Wilhelm Wundt (1832-1920)—this problem was "solved" by the doctrine of "psychophysical parallelism." In psychoanalysis, the same problem appeared in the form of "hysteria" or "conversion hysteria," terms that denoted the allegedly mysterious transformation of psychical (mental) conflict into physical (bodily) disease. In my first book, *Pain and Pleasure: A Study of Bodily Feelings*, I made a tentative attempt to resolve the problem by showing that *feelings* are intrinsically subjective and, in that sense, real by definition.[29] Later, influenced by Mead, I came to adopt the view that there is no mind; that, like mental illness, the term "mind" is itself a metaphor; hence, that the mind cannot be healthy or sick; and that instead of thinking and speaking about minds as entities, we ought to think and speak of selves, persons, and moral agents engaging in actions.[30]

Hayek versus Scientism

In my view, much of the importance of Hayek's work lies in his consistent and courageous opposition to scientific reductionism—which he called "scientism"—especially in his own field, economics. This aspect of Hayek's contribution to the cause of freedom is not sufficiently emphasized by libertarians. Ironically, Hayek himself did not fully appreciate its relevance to psychiatry and its role in illegitimizing the rationales for coercion under mental health auspices. Hayek's book, *The Counter-Revolution of Science* (1955), is an extended critique of scientism in the human "sciences." He wrote:

> The scientistic as distinguished from the scientific view is not an unprejudiced but a very prejudiced approach which, before it has considered its subject,

claims to know what is the most appropriate way of investigating it.... The social sciences in the narrower sense, i.e., those which used to be described as the "moral sciences," are concerned with man's conscious or reflected [sic] action, actions where a person can be said to choose between various courses open to him, and here the situation is essentially different [from the situation in the physical sciences].[31]

Albeit in rather convoluted prose, Hayek here restates the common sense distinction between action, choice, and decision on the one hand, and happening, event, and occurrence, on the other. On the plus side, Hayek deserves our admiration for his forthright criticism of the applications of mathematical economics to the great questions of social policy that form the ground on which economic relations rest. In an interview, he commented: "I don't want to be unkind to my old friend, the late Oskar Morgenstern, but while I think his book [*Theory of Games and Economic Behavior* by Oskar Morgenstern and John von Neumann[32]] is a great mathematical achievement, the first chapter which deals with economics is just wrong. I don't think that game theory has really made an important contribution to economics, but it's a very interesting mathematical discipline."[33]

On December 10, 1974, the evening before the Nobel ceremonies, Hayek delivered the Banquet address. In it, and in his Nobel acceptance speech the following day, Hayek reaffirmed his conviction that economics is not a true science. He courageously stated that the establishment of a Nobel Prize in Economics creates the false impression that economics is a science: "Now that the Nobel Memorial Prize for economic science has been created, one can only be profoundly grateful for having been selected as one of its joint recipients.... *Yet I must confess that if I had been consulted whether to establish a Nobel Prize in economics, I should have decidedly advised against it.*" He would have done so, he continued, because he feared that,

the Nobel Prize confers on an individual an authority which in economics no man ought to possess. This does not matter in the natural sciences. Here the influence exercised by an individual is chiefly an influence on his fellow experts; and they will soon cut him down to size if he exceeds his competence. But the influence of the economist that mainly matters is an influence over laymen: politicians, journalists, civil servants and the public generally.... I am not sure that it is desirable to strengthen the influence of a few individual economists by such a ceremonial and eye-catching recognition of achievements, perhaps of the distant past. I am therefore almost inclined to suggest that you require from your laureates an oath of humility, a sort of Hippocratic oath, never to exceed in public pronouncements the limits of their competence.

Or you ought at least, on conferring the prize, remind the recipient of the sage counsel of one of the great men in our subject, Alfred Marshall, who wrote: "Students of social science, must fear popular approval: Evil is with them when all men speak well of them."[34]

In his Nobel Prize Lecture, revealingly entitled "The pretense of knowledge"—a summary statement of his critique of scientism, first formulated in 1942 and set forth in detail in his 1955 book, *The Counter-Revolution of Science*—Hayek expanded on this theme. He stated:

[T]he still recent establishment of the Nobel Memorial Prize in Economic Science marks a significant step in the process by which, in the opinion of the general public, economics has been conceded some of the dignity and prestige of the physical sciences.... We have indeed at the moment little cause for pride: as a profession we have made a mess of things. It seems to me that this failure of the economists to guide policy more successfully is closely connected with their *propensity to imitate as closely as possible the procedures of the brilliantly successful physical sciences—an attempt which in our field may lead to outright error.* It is an approach which has come to be described as the "scientistic" attitude—an attitude which, as I defined it some thirty years ago, "is decidedly unscientific in the true sense of the word, since it involves a mechanical and uncritical application of habits of thought to fields different from those in which they have been formed."

After emphasizing that the sorts of information upon which economists base their explanations are not susceptible to mathematical treatment, Hayek continued:

What I mainly wanted to bring out by the topical illustration is that certainly in my field, but I believe also generally *in the sciences of man, what looks superficially like the most scientific procedure is often the most unscientific, and, beyond this, that in these fields there are definite limits to what we can expect science to achieve.* This means that to entrust to science—or to deliberate control according to scientific principles—more than scientific method can achieve may have deplorable effects.... *But it is by no means only in the field of economics that far-reaching claims are made on behalf of a more scientific direction of all human activities and the desirability of replacing spontaneous processes by "conscious human control." If I am not mistaken, psychology, psychiatry and some branches of sociology, not to speak about the so-called philosophy of history, are even more affected by what I have called the scientistic prejudice, and by specious claims of what science can achieve.* If we are to safeguard the reputation of science, and to prevent the arrogation of knowledge based on a superficial similarity of procedure with that of the physical sciences, much effort will have to be directed toward debunking such arrogations, some of which have by now become the vested interests of established university departments.... *The recognition of the insuperable limits to his knowledge ought indeed to teach the student of society a lesson of humility which should guard him against becoming an accomplice in men's fatal striving to control society—a striving which makes him not only a tyrant over his fellows, but which may well make him the destroyer of a civilization which no brain has designed but which has grown from the free efforts of millions of individuals.*[35]

These eloquent words call only for applause. I want to note only that Hayek's examples of scientisms include psychology and psychiatry; and that, from a political point of view, psychiatry is the single most important instance of scientism in America today.[36]

Conclusion

Hayek's well-founded insistence that, in a free society, laws must promulgate abstract or general rules is itself enough to invalidate the justification for all psychiatric coercions and excuses. We regulate the (mis)behavior of the "mentally healthy" person according to the criteria of guilt and innocence, but regulate the (mis)behavior of the "mentally sick" person according to the criteria of "diagnosis," "dangerousness," and "treatment."

Ostensibly, the mentally ill person is judged by a more elevated moral code than the mentally healthy person: he is excused from the harsh punishments of the criminal law and instead is treated with compassion and medical care. Actually, precisely by being so treated, he is "therapeutically" transformed—"for his own good"—into an object or thing. In effect, he is existentially murdered, leaving behind a nonperson, epitomized by the mental patient successfully cured by lobotomy.

12

Murray N. Rothbard

Murray N. Rothbard (1926-1995) was born and lived in New York except for a part of the year during the last decade of his life, when he was a professor of economics at the University of Nevada in Las Vegas. He was trained as an economist and was a devoted, but independent-minded, disciple of Mises. From the early fifties until his death, Rothbard was one of the most influential defenders of the philosophy of libertarianism. Widely regarded as holding "extreme" views, he was, like Mises, a pariah in academic circles.

In a commemorative essay, Llewellyn H. Rockwell, Jr.—founder and president of the Ludwig von Mises Institute in Auburn, Alabama and editor of the daily news site, "Lewrockwell.com"—hailed Rothbard as a man who "inspired a world-wide renewal in the scholarship of liberty. During 45 years of research and writing, in 25 books and thousands of articles, he battled every destructive trend in this century—socialism, statism, relativism, and scientism—and awakened a passion for freedom in thousands of scholars, journalists, and activists." Rockwell's essay is a fine summary of Rothbard's work. The following is a brief excerpt:

> Rothbard led the renaissance of the Austrian School of economics. He galvanized an academic and popular fight for liberty and property, against the omnipotent state and its court intellectuals.... Rothbard attended Mises's seminar at New York University from its first meeting, and became the student who would defend and extend Mises's ideas, push the Austrian School tradition to new heights, and integrate it with political theory.... Throughout history, the power elite has found profitable uses for the state. Rothbard never passed up a chance to name them, to explain how they did it, and to show how their actions harmed everyone else in society. Conflict was the central theme of Rothbardian political economy: the state vs. voluntary associations, and the struggle over the ownership and control of property...defense of capitalism, Rothbard was uncompromising. But he did not see the market as the be-all and end-all of the social order.... Like Mises, Rothbard gave up money and fame in academic economics to promote what is true and right.[1]

I have long maintained that the subject matter of psychiatry is conflict, not disease. Rockwell's reminder that "conflict was the central theme of Rothbardian political economy" reinforces the soundness of my suggestion, earlier in this book, that economics and psychiatry are similar, symmetrical disciplines.

Rothbard and Psychiatry

In February 2002, I published a short essay in *Liberty* entitled "Mises and psychiatry."[2] Shortly afterward, Rothbard's 1962 review of my book, *The Myth of Mental Illness*, originally prepared as "A Memo for the Volker Fund,"[3] appeared on the Llewellyn Rockwell website.[4] Two days later, the Rockwell website reprinted Rothbard's Keynote Address, "Psychoanalysis as a weapon," delivered at a symposium at the State University of New York in Albany, celebrating my sixtieth birthday in 1980.[5]

I shall refrain from speculating about why these pieces reappeared at this time. It is clear, or so it seems to me, that psychiatry sits uneasily in the belly of libertarianism. Rothbard wrote the review before we knew each other and before he became more familiar with my views. He praised the book as "a highly original and unique work...scattered throughout are intriguing libertarian points...attacks on governmental responsibility for inflation, on progressive income tax, on exploitation of one group by another, on totalitarianism, and on infringement of civil liberties, particularly in the practice of compulsory commitment of the (non-criminal) 'mentally ill.'" Approvingly, he acknowledged: "There is also certainly much value in criticizing the prevalent use of the cliché of 'mental illness' and the consequent linkage with somatic medicine. There are precious-few books on psychiatry, furthermore, which refer to Hayek's *Constitution of Liberty* or to Popper's *Poverty of Historicism*."

"Yet, despite these merits," Rothbard continued, "the book must be set down as an overall failure, for the bulk of the book consists in the setting forth of Szasz' own positive theories, which must be considered totally erroneous.... Szasz tosses out the crucial concepts of 'consciousness' and the 'unconscious.'... There are many weird results of this: one is that the crucial philosophic-psychologic concepts of individual will, responsibility, the line between the willed and the unwilled, etc. are tossed away...."

Criticizing my views on religion, Rothbard added: "Furthermore, in a fashion rather reminiscent of Ayn Rand, Dr. Szasz is almost fanatically anti-religion, and especially anti-Christian. Religion...[is] held to be responsible for a large part of the world's neuroses, for fostering 'childish dependency,' as well as for encouraging behavior not proper to man's life: e.g., humility, meekness, naiveté, etc., all of which add up, in Szasz' view, to 'incompetence.'"

The Myth of Mental Illness, Rothbard concluded, "eliminates the whole problem of moral responsibility for actions because it eliminates the whole problem of whether an act is consciously willed or decided upon, or not.... Szasz' fundamental philosophic error, perhaps, is his deliberate overthrowing of thinking in terms of 'entities' and 'substances,' i.e. 18th-century, natural-law, Aristotelian thinking."

Rothbard's criticism—epitomized by the charge that my argument "eliminates the whole problem of moral responsibility for actions"—was not merely erroneous, it stood the thesis of the book on its head. Rothbard blamed me for a feature intrinsic to the idea of mental illness and to the psychiatric coercions and excuses it justifies—precisely the errors and evils I attacked. My principal objective in writing *The Myth of Mental Illness* was to demonstrate that "mental illness" is not a medical disease, and to deligitimize its use as a weapon in the war that psychiatry, supported by the state, was waging against the individual, exemplified by the incarceration of innocent persons, justified as "hospitalization" and "treatment."

In his subsequent writings on psychiatry, Rothbard expressed unqualified agreement with my critique of the therapeutic state and the pivotal role of psychiatry in it. In his book, *For a New Liberty* (1978), he included a three-page section titled "Compulsory Commitment," devoted almost entirely to applauding my efforts to abolish involuntary psychiatric interventions:

- In the last decade, the libertarian psychiatrist and psychoanalyst Dr. Thomas S. Szasz has carried on a one-man crusade, at first seemingly hopeless but now increasingly influential, in the psychiatric field against compulsory commitment.[6]

- The libertarian Dr. Thomas Szasz has almost single-handedly managed to free many citizens from involuntary commitment...[7]

- One of the most shameful areas of involuntary servitude in our society is the widespread practice of compulsory commitment, or involuntary hospitalization, of mental patients.... To call this process "therapy" or "rehabilitation" is surely a cruel mockery of these terms.[8]

In his 1980 Keynote Address in Albany, Rothbard praised my efforts to defend individual liberty and personal responsibility against the threat posed to these values by psychiatry. He wrote:

> Thomas Szasz is justly honored for his gallant and courageous battle against the compulsory commitment of the innocent in the name of "therapy" and humanitarianism. But I would like to focus tonight on a lesser-known though corollary struggle of Szasz: against the use of psychoanalysis as a weapon to dismiss and dehumanize people, ideas, and groups that the analyst doesn't happen to like. Rather than criticize or grapple with the ideas or actions of people on their own terms, as correct or incorrect, right or wrong, good or bad, they are explained away by the analyst as caused by some form of neurosis. They are the ideas or actions of neurotic, or "sick," people.[9]

This brings us finally to the issue of religion. In the West, we no longer live in theocratic states. We live, as I have argued for forty years, in therapeutic states. We give medical, not religious, explanations for human behaviors (if we deem them bad, but not otherwise); and we justify the routine psychiatric imprisonment of innocent persons on medical, not religious, grounds. If those explanations and justifications are erroneous and invalid, as I maintain they are, then they are erroneous and invalid regardless of a person's religious belief or unbelief.

Conclusions

Rothbard had many fine qualities but did not lack for foibles. One of which was a fear of traveling (which he eventually overcame), another was his deceiving himself into believing that the fear was a "phobia" that constituted a "mental illness," and a third was that he submitted himself to Nathaniel Branden for "treatment." I present a brief account of this sad affair elsewhere in this volume.[10]

Rothbard's "travel phobia" appears to have been a relatively minor aspect of his health problems. He was also seriously overweight, probably suffered from coronary heart disease, and had a "phobia" of doctors. During the last year or two of his life, Rothbard felt increasingly weak and unwell. Instead of seeking help from a reputable New York cardiologist, Rothbard "consulted a doctor he had seen on a talk-show, whose *shtick* was that hospitals were giving far too many tests to patients, and that most of these procedures were unnecessary. His views fed into Rothbard's general suspicion of doctors."[11] He went to another doctor, who "suggested that he go Roosevelt Hospital, but Rothbard was adamantly opposed."[12] In a letter to Williamson Evers, he wrote: "I believe that doctors are, by and large, a group of highly paid butchers and murderers..."[13]

Highly paid compared to whom? Basketball players? Football coaches? Rock stars? Being highly paid is an odd charge against physicians coming from an arch defender of hard work and capitalism. Rothbard, much like Hayek, was naive about illness and medicine and avoided competent medical care—odd behaviors by two of the leading libertarian economists of our day.

On January 7, 1995, Rothbard collapsed and died of, biographer Justin Raimondo says, "heart failure." More likely, he died as a result of myocardial infarction.

One of the besetting sins of psychiatry and psychoanalysis and all so-called mental health professions is that, as Rothbard himself observed, instead of criticizing and grappling "with the ideas or actions of people on their own terms, as correct or incorrect, right or wrong, good or bad, they are explained away by the analyst." Sadly, this sin is not limited to psychoanalysts. All human beings are susceptible to it, libertarians included. Attributing embarrassing ideas and practices to mental illness is not the only way to avoid dealing with them. Ignoring them and refusing to take a stand about them is just as effective.

The Myth of Mental Illness was intended to be more than just an academic exercise in semantics. It was also intended to be a denunciation of the moral legitimacy of the most violent method that the modern state possesses and wields in its perpetual effort to domesticate and control people, namely, depriving innocent individuals—with the full support of physicians and lawyers—not only of liberty but virtually of all of their constitutional rights, in the name of helping them.

13

Robert Nozick

Robert Nozick (1938-2002)—philosopher, university professor at Harvard, and libertarian celebrity—presented himself as a man of wide-ranging interests. "Over the years," wrote Christopher Lehmann-Haupt in his *New York Times* obituary, Nozick "taught courses jointly with members of the government, psychology and economics departments, and at the divinity and law schools."[1] In his books, Nozick regularly cites psychiatrists, psychologists, psychoanalysts, and sociologists. In 1998, the American Psychological Association honored him with its Presidential Citation.

Because in this book I focus on the opinions of libertarians regarding deprivations of liberty under psychiatric auspices, their familiarity with psychiatry is relevant to judging their views. Academic specialists cannot be expected to be knowledgeable about social practices far afield from their areas of interest. But Nozick presented himself as a Renaissance man. And given his familiarity with the mental health field, he cannot have been unaware of the horrors of psychiatric slavery.

Anarchy, State, and Utopia

Libertarians generally regard the government as a bottomless source of political mendacity. Psychiatry is, and has always been, an arm of the government: it is authorized by the state to imprison individuals deemed mentally diseased and dangerous to themselves or others. Nevertheless, some libertarians do not regard the pronouncements of these agents of the state as a source of mendacity at all. To the contrary, they embrace them as scientific truths. Robert Nozick was such a libertarian.

Anarchy, State, and Utopia, published in 1974, was Nozick's first book and the basis for his being identified as a libertarian. In the Preface, he writes: "With reluctance, I found myself becoming convinced of (as they are so often called) libertarian views.... My earlier reluctance is not

163

present, because it has disappeared."[2] As we shall see, Nozick's reluctance about being identified as a libertarian soon returns with a vengeance.

The purpose of his book, Nozick states, is to examine "the nature of the state, its legitimate functions and its justifications."[3] One of the most important functions of the American state during Nozick's life was protecting people from themselves—a task the state accomplished by means of drug prohibition, suicide prohibition, and mental health laws, welded into a wide-ranging system of preventive detention and punishment, called "psychiatric diagnosis," "psychiatric hospitalization," and "psychiatric treatment." One of the leading professional organizations fueling, justifying, and profiting from the government's wars on drugs and mental illness is the American Psychological Association. Nozick's receiving the Association's 1998 Presidential Citation must be seen in that context.

Despite his stated aim for *Anarchy, State, and Utopia*, Nozick never even mentions drug use and drug laws, mental illness, civil commitment, the insanity defense, or suicide. Yet, references to Erving Goffman and Helmut Schoeck are evidence of his familiarity with these subjects.[4] Goffman, author of *Asylums* (1961),[5] was a co-founder—with George Alexander and myself—of the American Association for the Abolition of Involuntary Mental Hospitalization in 1971.[6] Schoeck, an influential sociologist-philosopher, was the co-editor of *Psychiatry and Responsibility* (1962), to which I contributed a chapter on "Psychiatry as a Social Institution."[7]

Anarchy, State, and Utopia is full of remarks with obvious implications for psychiatric practice. For example, Nozick writes: "If anything, there is a stronger case for nonaggression among individuals...."[8] The libertarian nonaggression principle is irreconcilable with coercive-paternalistic psychiatric practices. Although silent about psychiatry's wars against masturbation, homosexuality, drug abuse, mental illness, and suicide, Nozick declares: "My nonpaternalistic position holds that someone may choose (or permit another) to do to himself *anything*, unless he has acquired an obligation to some third party not to do or allow it."[9] Nozick never acknowledges that his professed adherence to this principle logically makes him a deadly enemy of psychiatric principles and practices and is inconsistent with his uncritical references to the works of mental health professionals.

Nozick says that he opposes preventive detention, which he describes as "encompass[ing] imprisoning someone, not for any crime he has committed, but because it is predicted of him that the probability is significantly higher than normal that he will commit a crime."[10] By using the passive voice—"it is predicted"—Nozick manages to avoid mentioning that it is psychiatrists and psychologists who do such predicting. Instead of offering a single concrete example of preventive detention—exemplified by civil commitment—Nozick fills page after page with tortured prose, such as the following: "But if the evil (it is feared) the person may do really does hinge upon decisions for wrong which he has not yet made, then the earlier principles will rule preventive detention or restraint illegitimate and impermissible."[11]

Nozick fails to stand up and be counted for the libertarian principles he professes to support. Instead, like the lamentable animal-rights activist Peter Singer, Nozick speculates at length about the rights of animals and the morality of eating them. "Animals," he pontificates, "count for something..... Given that animals are to count for something, is the extra gain obtained by eating them rather than nonanimal products greater than the moral cost? How might these questions be decided?"[12]

Nozick mentions eating animals but conveniently ignores the myriad moral problems we might project into the other uses of animals and animal products, in agriculture and transportation, clothing and household goods, as pets, guides, rescue animals, subjects of medical experiments, sources of vaccines, and as body parts for preventing and treating human diseases.[13]

Nozick asserts that we ought to accord rights to animals. He does not say that we ought to accord rights to persons psychiatrists diagnose as mentally ill. His compassionate agonizing about the rights of animals, combined with his cold-hearted acceptance of the status of mental patients as objects devoid of rights, is symptomatic of his deep-seated protectionist-statist impulses, evident in his subsequent works.

Philosophical Explanations

In 1981, Nozick published *Philosophical Explanations*, a tome weighing in at 764 pages. He comments on many recondite subjects and offers fantastic speculations, more likely to impress or put off the reader than to inform him. For example, he devotes two pages to a discussion of mathematician George Cantor's ideas about diagonal numbers, real numbers, and positive integers.[14] There are not many non-mathematicians who can understand what Nozick has to say on this subject.

It is not that Nozick shies away from making observations about the workings of the human mind. For example, he offers this science-fiction fantasy about sleeping, dreaming, and "the identity of the self": "Some writers have speculated that when people sleep and dream, an astral body actually moves off from the sleeping body and in some realm performs the dreamed action."[15]

Nozick's discussion of free will is similarly obtuse. He declares: "My concern with free will, however, *is not rested* [sic] *in a desire to punish people or hold them responsible, or even to be held responsible myself.*"[16] The concept of free will implies responsibility and the options of punishing or forgiving persons for actions we deem to be bad or criminal. According to psychiatric-legal doctrine, mentally healthy persons have free will and deserve to be punished for the crimes they commit, whereas "severely" mentally ill persons ("psychotics") lack free will and deserve to be "treated" for the mental diseases that *caused* them to commit crimes. I emphasize this elementary point because experts on the mind regularly attribute impairment or loss of free will to mental illness, with disastrous consequences for the "patient."

Nozick's avoidance of addressing the intimate connections between responsibility and psychiatry was deliberate. He contributed a long chapter on the subject to a multi-author book on philosophy without even mentioning mental health laws or policies. Instead, this is the sort of thing he says about responsibility:

- That being coerced into not doing act A is not a sufficient condition for being unfree to do A is shown by the following example: You threaten to get me fired from my job if I do A, and I refrain from doing A because of this threat and am coerced into not doing A. However, unbeknownst to me you are bluffing...[17]

- P threatens to do something if Q does A (and P knows he is making this threat). This threat renders Q's doing A substantially less eligible as a course of conduct than not doing A.[18]

Ludwig von Mises—a serious scholar and committed anticommunist as well as anti-Nazi—was an academic pariah. Robert Nozick—a professor who could "range[s] copiously over relativity theory and quantum theory, cosmology, modal logic, topology, evolutionary biology, neuroscience, cognitive psychology, decision theory, economics, and even Soviet history" (Colin McGinn)—was an academic superstar. Libertarians who admire or cite his work do so, I fear, more because they are dazzled by the reflected glory of the name "Harvard" and hope it will deflect onto libertarianism generally, than because of the worth of Nozick's contributions to the philosophy of liberty and responsibility. In my opinion, discoursing about personal responsibility and ignoring psychiatry is like discussing the Civil War and ignoring slavery. Perhaps this is what is expected of a Harvard philosopher nowadays. The noted English sociologist David Martin cogently observes: "Such is the state of contemporary philosophy, many of the really serious human issues have to be handled by theology."[19] Sadly, the connection between responsibility and psychiatry is too hot even for theology to touch.

Nozick refers approvingly to the authoritarian-coercive Austrian psychiatrist Viktor Frankl.[20] He does not mention that Frankl endorsed and engaged in psychiatry's most loathsome practices, including lobotomy, which, although not a neurosurgeon, he himself performed.[21] He proudly wrote: "I have signed *authorizations* for lobotomies without having cause to regret it. In a few cases, *I have even carried out transorbital lobotomy.* However, I promise you that the human dignity of our patients is not violated in this way.... What matters is not the technique or therapeutic approach as such, be it drug treatment or shock treatment, but the spirit in which it is being carried out."[22] To boot, Frankl's claim of having been an inmate at Auschwitz appears to be open to doubt. Raul Hilberg, one of the founding fathers of Holocaust research, brackets Victor Frankl's *Man's Search for Meaning* with Benjamin Wilkomirski's infamous *Memoirs*[23] and states: "The approximate dating of his [Frankl's] stays in Theresienstadt and Auschwitz is deducible from the [his] book.... The ghetto museum of Theresienstadt could find no records of Frankl's arrival and departure."[24]

The Examined Life

In 1989, Nozick published *The Examined Life: Philosophical Meditations*, a collection of twenty-seven essays on subjects ranging from creativity, to evil, happiness, the Holocaust, and love. This book leaves no doubt about Nozick's extensive familiarity with psychiatry. He refers respectfully to the ideas of Sigmund Freud, Erik Erikson, Abraham Maslow, and David Shapiro, and even cites the latter's technical text, *Neurotic Styles*.[25]

The Examined Life is Nozick's most personal work, and a curious book it is. In the Introduction, he declares that he wants to set the record straight: *he is not a libertarian and does not want to identified as a libertarian*: "We do not want to get committed to any one particular understanding or locked into it. This danger looms large for writers; in the public's mind or in their own they easily can become identified with a particular 'position.' Having myself written earlier a book of political philosophy that marked out a distinctive view, one that now seems seriously inadequate to me...I am especially aware of the difficulty of living down an intellectual past or escaping it."[26]

The first chapter of *The Examined Life* is titled "Dying." After several pages of trivia couched in the rhetoric of uplift, Nozick proposes "the extreme speculation, that in death a person's organized energy—some might say spirit—becomes the governing structure of a new universe that *bubbles out orthogonally* right there and then from the event of *her* death. The nature of the new universe created then will be determined by the level of reality, stability, serenity, etc., that she has managed to reach in her lifetime. And perhaps she then continues eternally as that kind of God [sic] of that universe."[27] Nozick calls this a "speculation." I call it self-indulgent nonsense. Nozick says that his fictitious energy bubbles up at a right angle, but he doesn't say at a right angle to what.

At the end of the chapter on "Dying," Nozick remarks: "I understand the urge to cling to life until the very end, yet I find another course more appealing." Is he about to broach the subject of rational suicide? Of the psychiatric prohibition of suicide and its punishment by civil commitment? Heavens, no. To the contrary, befitting his communitarian identity, he recommends hastening the end of one's life by *risking it for others:* "After an ample life, a person who still possesses energy, acuity, and decisiveness might choose to seriously risk his life or lay it down for another person or for some noble and decent cause."

Glorifying Gandhi and Martin Luther King as icons of near-divine nobility, Nozick enthuses: "Utilizing the freedom of action that is gained by the willingness to run serious risks, people's ingenuity will devise new modes and patterns of effective action which others can emulate, individually or jointly...some might seriously weigh spending their penultimate years in a brave and noble endeavor to benefit others...not going gentle into the good night or raging against the dying of the light but, near the end, shining their light most brightly."[28] Good people don't wait until they are dying before they try to benefit others.

The Examined Life and Suicide

Socrates, whom we credit with the phrase "the unexamined life is not worth living," killed himself. Camus, a philosopher of real life, not airy nothings, declared that suicide is the only "truly serious philosophical problem."[29] Nozick finds no room in his philosophy for suicide. He does find room in it, as befits a liberal-statist academic, for the practice that even philosophers, who ought to know better, misleadingly call "physician-assisted suicide" (PAS).

In 1996, Compassion in Dying—a private, nonprofit organization established by wealthy donors, ostensibly to help "dying patients" end their lives when they want to—brought suit against the state of Washington, seeking a declaration by the court that the statutes that prohibit "causing or aiding another person to commit suicide violate the Federal Constitution."[30] Actually, the organization was a front to increase the powers and privileges of physicians, especially psychiatrists.[31]

Lawyers for the physicians of four dying patients claimed that the doctors have a constitutionally protected right to "assist" terminally ill suicidal patients by giving them a prescription for a lethal drug; that terminally ill patients have a constitutionally protected right to receive PAS; and that PAS is a *bona fide* medical treatment. The same claim was advanced in another the case, known as *Quill v. Vacco*, where the plaintiffs declared: "[Writing] a prescription [for a lethal drug], which only a licensed medical doctor can provide...*is a complex medical task*."[32]

As I show in *Fatal Freedom*, the term "physician-assisted suicide" is at once an oxymoron and a Trojan horse, seemingly helping the cause of liberty but actually harming it.[33] The program to promote PAS is but one instance in the relentlessly growing practice of the medicalization of life. The supporters of PAS claim that their aim is to increase "patient autonomy." However, the policy they propose adds the power to provide "suicide" to the physicians' power to prevent it. The practical consequences of making PAS contingent on psychiatric approval are similar to the consequences of making sex change operations contingent on psychiatric approval: it is an invitation to involuntary psychiatric intervention, illustrated by the repeated psychiatric incarceration of the respected libertarian economist, Deirdre (Donald) McCloskey.[34]

Coercive suicide prevention is to psychiatric slavery as the fugitive slave laws were to chattel slavery. The slave owner was determined to prevent his slave's self-determined escape from slavery, except on his, the master's, terms (by manumission). The psychiatrist is determined to prevent his patient's self-determined escape from life, except on his, the doctor's, terms (by prescription). Each regards the Other's autonomy as the rejection of his, the "benefactor's," authority—the ultimate offense (sin, crime, mental illness). It is important to emphasize here that while Nozick approved PAS, he avoided considering, much less approving, physician-unassisted suicide, that is, *suicide without psychiatric permission.*

Along with the ACLU and other liberal-statist organizations, a group of philosophers submitted an *amicus curiae* brief to the Supreme Court supporting the suit for legalized PAS. The philosophers' panel was headed by the influential anti-libertarian Ronald Dworkin and included Harvard philosopher John Rawls, whose views Nozick opposed in *Anarchy, the State, and Utopia*. The philosophers' brief, prepared by Dworkin, began with a *powerful endorsement of coercive psychiatric suicide prevention*: "[The panel recognizes] that people may make such momentous decisions impulsively or out of *emotional depression*... States have a constitutionally legitimate interest in *protecting individuals from irrational...unstable decisions to hasten their own death*."[35] This was the group and the brief that Nozick joined.

The philosophers then registered their opposition to "*forcing* a competent dying patient to live in agony a few weeks longer,"[36] asserted their inability to discern significant differences between refusing treatment and receiving PAS, and concluded: "[D]eclaring that terminally ill patients in great pain do not have a constitutional right *to control their own deaths*, even in principle, seems alien to our constitutional system."[37] In June 1997, the United State Supreme Court, by a vote of 9 to 0, upheld state laws prohibiting assisted suicide.[38]

The Unexamined Life

The correct title for *The Examined Life* would have been *The Unexamined Life*. After approvingly citing "methods of achieving enlightenment" in the "Eastern tradition,"[39] Nozick offers this gem about sexual intercourse (presumably heterosexual, although he does not say): "[I]n sex one also can engage in metaphysical exploration, knowing the body and person of another as a map or microcosm of the very deepest reality, a clue to its nature and purpose."[40] This perspective on the sex act as a metaphysical rather than physical exploration raises the romanticization of coitus to a cosmic level. In its fatuous exaggeration of the importance and glories of the sex act Nozick's view of the sex act resembles Nathaniel Branden's as "the ultimate form in which man experiences *perceptually* that he is good and that life is good."[41]

It gets worse. Nozick endorses the idea of "motiveless action." He writes: "The *Bhagavad-Gita* speaks of action, by which I think it means making oneself a pure and impersonal vehicle *through which something else can act* and be transmitted."[42] Nozick's laudatory reference to the *Bhagavad-Gita*—an ancient Indian mystical text written in Sanskrit—implies that having motives for actions renders the actor an impure vehicle, which contradicts Nozick's idealization of the altruistic actor, touted elsewhere in the book. I don't have to speculate about what a motiveless action is. I know what it is: an oxymoron that also happens to be an indispensable legal-psychiatric fiction and strategy. Nozick's "pure" motiveless actor is but another version of the psychiatrist's "legally-medically innocent" murderous madman who is "pure"—not responsible for his act, an automaton "through which something else can act." The psychiatrist calls that something else: *irresistible impulses, voices, delusions, schizophrenia, psychosis*, in short, *exculpatory criminal insanity.*

In a chapter tellingly titled "The Zigzag of Politics," Nozick not only distances himself from his earlier libertarianism, he apologizes for it: "The libertarian position I once propounded now seems to me seriously inadequate, in part because it did not fully knit the humane considerations and joint cooperative activities more closely into its fabric. There are some things we choose to do together, through government in our solemn marking of our human solidarity."[43]

I believe this is a thoroughly confused and mistaken view. Strictly speaking, we cannot *choose* to do anything "through government": inherent in the idea of government is the delegation of choice from private persons to political representatives qua public authorities. The delegation of choice may be tacit, as in a devout Catholic's submission to the Church, or explicit, as in a voter's casting a ballot for his "representative." In any case, an essential function or result of government is limitation of choice by the individual.

It is an illusion that we "choose" to fight an enemy "together." Given the diverse population of modern nation states, there are always many people who do not share the majority's view even of the identity of the enemy, let alone the necessity of fighting him. The war on drugs is but one obvious example.

As I see it, libertarianism is a political philosophy, the ideology of the minimalist state, summed up in the adage, "he who governs least, governs best." In short, libertarianism is the philosophy of individual liberty and personal responsibility, embedded in and fostered by a political system that maximizes the scope of personal self-control and minimizes the role of external coercion. To put it more picturesquely, libertarianism is the ethic of the swimmer, the needs of non-swimmers provided primarily by families, private philanthropies, religious groups, and other informal, charitable organizations. The state is the lifeguard of last resort, prohibited from "saving" individuals who are not drowning, let alone who are not even at the beach. Communitarianism, in contrast, is the ethic of the lifeguard, with everyone viewed as an actual or potential drowning person in need of lifesaving intervention. Nozick is a communitarian-utilitarian. He repeats the conventional liberal slander against libertarianism, that it lacks compassion:

> The libertarian view looked solely at the purpose of government, not at its *meaning*...if helping those in *need*, as compared to further bettering of those already well off, counts as relationally more intense and enduring from *our* side and from the side of the receivers also, then the relational stance can explain what puzzles utilitarianism, *viz.*, why a concern for bettering others' situation concentrates especially upon the needy. If manna descended from heaven to improve the situation of the needy, all without our aid, we would have to find another way to jointly express and intensify our relational ties.[44]

Only an individual can "aid" Peter without coercing Paul. The state can "aid" Peter only by coercing Paul. Moreover, the state often "aids" Peter by coercing him, as in the case of psychiatric "help." These passages may explain, in part, why Nozick remained silent about psychiatric slavery, modernity's model of helping the needy[45]—because he approved of it.

Toward the end of *The Examined Life*, Nozick expresses concern about his views being "vulgarized," and makes an unusual, and unusually narcissistic, request of the reader: "Since wide-scale distortions get based upon secondary descriptions, there is one precaution I can take: to ask that no reader summarize this book's contents or present slogans or catchwords from it, no school give examinations on the material it contains."[46]

The Nature of Rationality and *Invariances*

Although rationality and irrationality are key psychiatric concepts, in *The Nature of Rationality* (1993) Nozick makes no reference to psychiatry, abnormal behavior, irrationality, insanity, mental illness, psychosis, and psychopathology.[47] I do not understand how rationality can be analyzed without reference to irrationality, and vice versa. Nozick does: he treats rationality as a philosophical subject, distinct and separate from irrationality, which he ignores. Does he do this because he regards irrationality as belonging to mental illness, and regards mental illness as a disease like malaria or melanoma, about which a professional philosopher must remain silent? Nozick does not tell us. What he does tell us is that he likes to dabble in psychoanalysis and is indifferent to the war on drugs.

After commenting on the familiar symbolic utility of "neurotic symptom," he adds: "I am not aware of a clear statement in the Freudian literature of this equation [of the symbolic and what it stands for] or of the weaker claim that *some* of the utility of what is symbolized is imputed back to the symbol, even though some such version is presupposed."[48] Nozick is profoundly ignorant about the vast psychoanalytic literature on the symbolic meaning of seemingly irrational behaviors, in the works, for example, of Adler, Jung, Rank, Sartre, and, of course, Freud. Nozick's remark is, moreover, evidence of his interest in the work of mental health professionals and hence of his obligation, as a moral philosopher, to take a stand on the issue of psychiatric slavery.

Nozick's tacit endorsement of drug prohibition confirms that he is a commmunitarian, not a libertarian. He writes: "On these grounds [of symbolic utility], one might claim that certain antidrug enforcement measures *symbolize* reducing the amount of drug use.... Simply halting the current action would deprive people of its symbolic utility, something they are unwilling to let happen."[49] This is an amoral justification for persecuting drug abusers. For whites, chattel slavery, for Nazis anti-Semitism, and for Communists anti-capitalism had "symbolic utility."

In his last book, *Invariances: The Structure of the Objective World* (2001), Nozick "looks at the nature of truth and objectivity...examines the function of subjective consciousness in an objective world," and discusses whether "truth in general is relative to culture and social factors."[50] Despite this wildly ambitious aim, he finds no room, in 416 pages of text, to consider matters related to psychiatry. He grandly concludes by acknowledging that "human behavior is complex; it is complexly caused, and that explains why we don't have *yet* a good theory of it."[51]

Conclusions

Literally, the term "philosophy" means love of wisdom. Nozick, professional philosopher, had no more interest in wisdom than the professional theologian has in understanding gods. He was interested in his "office," in the root sense of the term, as a socially authenticated position of authority regarding a branch of knowledge.

Perhaps in part because Nozick was a professor of philosophy at Harvard, many libertarians embraced him as one of their flag bearers. Since his death, he has been virtually sanctified as a philosophical genius. I do not share this judgment. My view of Nozick is closer to that of Colin McGinn, professor of philosophy at Rutgers. In a long review of Nozick's *Invariances* in *The New York Review of Books*, McGinn writes:

> Robert Nozick's intellectual energy is a thing of wonder. In *Invariances* he
> ranges copiously over relativity theory and quantum theory, cosmology, modal

logic, topology, evolutionary biology, neuroscience, cognitive psychology, decision theory, economics, and even Soviet history—not to mention his strictly philosophical forays into the nature of truth, objectivity, necessity, consciousness, and ethics.... Duly intimidated, thoroughly outclassed, reduced to silence, the reader may find himself brooding on his shortcomings."[52]

McGinn speaks of Nozick's "blabbering incoherence," exemplified by statements such as the following: "I suggest that *thoughts*, that is, linguistic or at any rate semantic items, are the *representations* of...parallel distributed processing neural states. Thoughts in words or wordlike entities are the way is which these PDP neural states present themselves to us.... Semantic content is *the way in which (certain) neural states feel to us.*"[53] McGinn comments: "Obviously, thoughts don't represent neural states in the sense of being about them...what could it mean to say that a thought about London, say, is just the way your neural states feel to you?"[54] Here and throughout much of his writing, Nozick commits the sin of what the French call "*il faut epater le bourgeois*" ("you must shock the bourgeois"), a sure sign of the intellectual poseur. Did Nozick understand relativity theory, quantum theory, and topology, or did his references to these subjects serve as ornamentations for his carefully crafted persona?

Harvard Philosophy Department Chair Christine Korsgaard hailed Nozick as "a brilliant and fearless thinker...apparently interested in everything."[55] Nozick wrote about everything, but I am not sure he was *interested* in anything. He wrote about death, without mentioning the psychiatric persecution of persons called "suicide risks"; about gay rights, without mentioning the long history of the psychiatric persecution of homosexuals; about drug use and drug laws, without mentioning the psychiatric persecution of persons stigmatized as "addicts"; and about political freedom and the state, without mentioning the wars on personal liberty and individual responsibility waged by psychiatric agents of the therapeutic state.

Nozick worked with many eminent academics who were members or friends of the mental health establishment. He participated in interdisciplinary groups charged with "studying compelling questions...that no single discipline or department has managed to answer alone." Among these subjects were "Substance Abuse" and "Drugs and Addictions," which he "studied" with such leading advocates of psychiatric savageries as Sally Satel.[56]

Nozick's attitude toward psychiatric coercions was like that of the three legendary Japanese monkeys' attitude toward wickedness: hear no evil, see no evil, and speak no evil. Wittgenstein famously said, "Whereof one cannot speak, thereof one must be silent." Nozick's motto might have been, "Whereof one cannot speak flatteringly, thereof one must not speak."

Qui tacet consentit. (He who remains silent consents.)

14

Julian Simon

Julian Simon (1932-1998) was professor of business administration at the University of Maryland and distinguished senior fellow at the Cato Institute. Dubbed "the doom-slayer" because of his irrefutable demonstration of the falsehoods of the liberal environmental doomsday industry, he is widely recognized as one of the most brilliant free-market economists of the second half of the twentieth century. Stephen Moore, director of fiscal policy studies at the Cato Institute, offered this summary of Simon's work:

> [In the 1970s and early 1980s], everyone knew that the world was headed to hell in a hand basket. We could see the signs right before our very eyes. We had just lived through a decade of gasoline lines, Arab oil embargoes, severe food shortages in the Third World, nuclear accidents, and raging global inflation.... The most famous declinist of the era, biologist Paul Ehrlich, had appeared on the Tonight Show with Johnny Carson to fill Americans with fear of impending world famine and make gloomy prognostications, such as, "If I were a gambler, I would bet even money that England will not exist in the year 2000."... [T]hanks to iconoclast Julian Simon, we now know that it was all so wrong.... He showed that, over time, the environment had been getting cleaner, not dirtier. He showed that the "population bomb" was a result of a massive global reduction in infant mortality rates and a stunning increase in life expectancy. "If we place value on human life," Simon argued, "then those trends are to be celebrated, not lamented." Simon's central premise was that people are the ultimate resource.... The ultimate embarrassment for the Malthusians was when Paul Ehrlich bet Simon $1,000 in 1980 that five resources (of Ehrlich's choosing) would be more expensive in 10 years. Ehrlich lost: 10 years later every one of the resources had declined in price by an average of 40 percent.[1]

In his professional role as economist, Simon showed no interest in psychiatry, mental illness, or mental health policy. However, in his role as a private person who felt depressed, he wrote a book, ambitiously titled *Good Mood: The New Psychology of Overcoming Depression.*[2]

It is an embarrassingly bad book, a naive and uninformed piece of pop psychology. However, Simon's well-justified eminence as a libertarian makes it necessary that I take note of it.

Simon's Psychology of Depression

Simon begins his book by defining depression in terms of how the subject feels: "Are you sad? Do you have a low opinion of yourself? Does a sense of helplessness and hopelessness weigh you down?"[3] Sadness, opinion, and a sense of helplessness or hopelessness are feelings, not diseases. Treating them *as if* they were diseases is an assumption, a leap of faith. Simon never says, in so many words, whether depression is or is not a disease. However, he consistently writes as if it were one, and naively supports his description-as-definition of it with ludicrous government propaganda: "Eighty percent of people with serious depression can be treated successfully. Medication or psychological therapies, or combinations of both, usually relieve symptoms in weeks."[4] This is precisely the kind of misinformation that, in the economic area, Simon mercilessly satirized. Yet, throughout his book, Simon speaks in this psychiatric jargon. Over and over again, we hear about "depression," "symptoms, "medication," "therapy," and "cure." The ideas, interventions, and terms never mentioned include "mental hospital," "involuntary mental hospitalization," "psychiatric coercion," "suicide," "suicide prevention," "psychiatric force and fraud." His "mathematical" model of depression is illustrative of the pseudoscientific, pop psychology style to which Simon sinks in this book:

$$\text{Mood} = \frac{(\text{Perceived state of oneself})}{(\text{Hypothetical benchmark state})}$$

Simon explains: "If the numerator (perceived state of oneself) in the Mood Ratio is low compared to the denominator (hypothetical benchmark state)—a situation which I'll call a Rotten Ratio—your mood will be bad."[5] And so it goes. Simon continues: "Now we are ready to ask: How can you manipulate your *mental apparatus* so as to reduce the flow of negative self-comparisons about which you feel helpless? There are several possibilities for any given person..."[6]

It is painful to read such gibberish coming from so brilliant a mind. Simon seems utterly unaware that people such as Mary Baker Eddy,

Emile Coué, Paul Dubois, and many others have plowed the same field and harvested the same worthless crop.[7] A few more examples of embarrassing banalities and "false facts" should suffice:

- "When you are depressed you *feel sad*..."[8] And when you are happy, you feel joyous.

- "Postpartum depression follows a whole series of biological changes and *seems to have no psychological* explanation."[9] It does not seem so to me. The idea that postpartum depression *might also be* a psychological reaction to the realization of enormous responsibilities entailed in becoming a mother does not seem to occur to Simon.

- "Strange as it may seem, a person sometimes gets enough benefits from her/his depression, so that the person prefers remaining depressed—despite all its unpleasantness—to being undepressed."[10] Simon is like a child who has discovered that the earth is not flat, even though it seems flat, and calls the insight "strange."

- "The device of 'counting your blessings' can be used to change your denominator, by changing the benchmark comparison that you make..."[11]

- Chapter heading: "Religious Conversion Can Cure Depression."[12]

Only toward the end of his book does Simon actually tell us something about what he calls his thirteen-year siege of severe depression. This is what he tells us:

- "My depression had its proximate cause in an event in 1962. I was then a businessman running my own new small business, and I did something that was morally wrong—not a big thing, but enough to throw me into the blackest depth of despair for more than a year, and then into an ongoing grey depression thereafter."[13] The reader cannot help but wonder what Simon's misdeed was.

- "I was surreptitiously operating on the nutty presumption that if I punished myself enough, no one else would punish me for my misdeed."[14] This is not a "nutty presumption." In religion, it is called "penance." Was publishing this book and hinting at his misdeed a part of Simon's penance?

- "All those years I concealed my depression so that *no one except my wife* knew about it."[15] If Simon was able to successfully hide his depression from everyone, including his children and colleagues, except his wife, perhaps he would have been able to hide it from her too, had he wanted to. Did he not want to? Was it, in part at least, a message to her?

- "An Orthodox Jewish friend of mine told me that it is one of the basic precepts of the Jewish Sabbath that one is not allowed to think about anything that will make him or her sad or anxious during that day. This struck me as an extraordinarily good idea and I tried to obey that rule."[16] It worked. Doubt about Simon's "illness" increases.

- "[My mother] never seemed satisfied with me as a child (though perhaps she really was). No matter how well I did something, she always urged that I could do better. Then this startling insight came to me: Why should I still pay attention to my mother's strictures?" This insight occurred to Simon in 1986, when he was fifty-four years old. It took him a long time to grow up.

Good Mood is devoid of evidence of familiarity with the complex history of the cure of souls, religious and psychiatric. Yet Simon calls it a "New Psychology of Overcoming Depression." It is as if a psychiatrist—who shows no evidence of ever having heard of Adam Smith, Frederic Bastiat, Vilfredo Pareto, Ludwig von Mises, Friedrich Hayek, John Maynard Keynes, or Murray Rothbard—were to write a book, subtitled a "New Method for Overcoming (Economic) Depression."

Simon's silence about the moral, legal, and political aspects of psychiatry deserves a brief comment. Silence is a kind of speech. It suggests that Simon agrees with the conventional psychiatric-legal view that "infants, idiots, and the insane" are not fit for liberty. This interpretation is supported by Simon's inviting Albert Ellis to write a Foreword for his book. Ellis is a psychologist, the inventor and promoter of Rational-Emotive Behavioral Therapy (REBT), and a firm believer in mental illness and involuntary mental hospitalization.[17]

Conclusion

"There is," remarked Sir Joshua Reynolds (1723-1792), the great English portrait painter, "no expedient to which man will not resort to avoid the real labor of thinking."[18] Although Simon reveled in the labor of real thinking about the economics and politics of ecology, he rejected critical thinking about the economics and politics of psychiatry. Albeit a self-declared libertarian, Simon ignored the vast apparatus of contemporary American psychiatric slavery. Perhaps it is worth mentioning that Simon was married to Rita J. Simon, a distinguished sociologist, university professor in the Department of Justice, Law, and Society in the School of Public Affairs at American University in Washington, D.C., former editor of the *American Sociological Review*, and the author and co-author of numerous books, among them a major study of the insanity defense.[19] She is a firm believer in mental illness and a zealous advocate of psychiatric coercions and excuses.[20]

Simon's fame rests on his skepticism about economic and sociological data, falsified to advance the ideological and political agenda of a biased class of "experts." He failed to entertain similar doubts about the authority of his mother and suffered a great deal of unhappiness largely as a result of it. His book *Good Mood*—in which he unashamedly displays his gullibility about psychiatry—diminishes his legacy.

15

Deirdre N. McCloskey

Henry Herbert, the Second Earl of Pembroke (1534-1601), famously declared, "A parliament can do any thing but make a man a woman, and a woman a man."[1] Little did the Earl suspect that his powerful metaphor about the political power of Parliament in sixteenth-century England would reappear as a controversial legal, medical, and political issue in twentieth-century America.

Transsexualism—the term and the "disease"—was invented in 1953, by Harry Benjamin, M.D., a German-born, American endocrinologist practicing in New York City. The transsexual person feels "trapped" in the body of the wrong sex and wishes to acquire the physical accouterments he or she does not possess. In this respect, the phenomenon differs from homosexuality and other sexual deviations classified as mental diseases. The endocrinological and surgical measures necessary to accomplish, or at least approximate, the transsexual's goal only became available in the twentieth century. This is how and why the elaborate machinery of "evaluating" the "suitability" of transsexuals for "treatment" by "sex reassignment surgery" and granting them permission for it became matters for psychiatric authorities to adjudicate and administer.

Crossing: From Donald to Deirdre McCloskey

"When we step into the family, by the act of being born," remarked Gilbert K. Chesterton, "we do step into a world which is incalculable, into a world which has its own strange laws, into a world which could do without us, into a world we have not made."[2] He might have added that, by the act of being born, we also step into a world that attributes to us certain roles and role obligations that are often difficult, and sometimes impossible, to fulfill, overcome, reject, or escape. One such role is our sexual identity, chromosomally determined at conception, and socially and legally defined at birth and after. This identity constitutes our most basic "contract" with our fellow man. I place the word "contract" between quotation marks because, literally, the term implies a voluntary agreement between two or more persons.

Departure from this basic contract—especially crossing the Iron Curtain between the sexes—disorients and disorders social relations: bisexuality, homosexuality, cross-dressing, and transsexualism disrupt the subject's relations to his parents, spouse, children, friends, and society. This is why each of these behaviors has at one time or another been prohibited and punished by religion, custom, law, and psychiatry.

Deirdre McCloskey—the Tinbergen Distinguished Professor at Erasmus University in Rotterdam, The Netherlands—is an internationally recognized economic historian, teacher, and writer. In addition to numerous works on economics, she is the author of *Crossing: A Memoir* (1999), an autobiographical account of her journey from Donald to Deirdre McCloskey.[3] What makes McCloskey's book of particular importance for the present study is that she is, to my knowledge, the only prominent libertarian who has been personally violated by psychiatrists. This circumstance lends special force to her views on the relations between libertarian philosophy and psychiatric practice.

Donald McCloskey was born in 1942 and had a seemingly normal childhood. He married, had a son and a daughter, and led the life of a well-adjusted, successful academic, teaching both history and economics at the University of Iowa.

When he reached puberty, McCloskey began to dress in women's clothes. In 1994, at the age of fifty-two, he decided that he was transsexual and began to take steps to become a woman. *Crossing* is a candid account of his transsexual odyssey. In the following summary, I cite primarily those aspects of the story that touch on the author's contacts with psychiatrists. Recalling her early cross-dressing years, McCloskey relates:

> As a teenager Donald broke into neighboring houses to wear the crinolines, and shoes that fit, and garter belts and all the equipment of a 1950s girl.... He was never caught...no one suspected, and the cross-dressing never became an issue. *Thank goodness,* thought Deirdre. In the 1950s they gave electroshock treatment for homosexuality, to say nothing of gender crossing. In later decades the psychiatrists persisted, and "gender identity disorder," as homosexuality was in the dark ages before 1973, is an item in the *Diagnostic and Statistical Manual of Mental Disorders,* fourth edition, the DSM-IV. The disorder did not appear in the DSM-IV until seven years after the psychiatrists guiltily removed homosexuality.[4]

Fifty-two years is a long time, the better part of a person's life span. During those years, his parents, siblings, wife, and children related to McCloskey as son, brother, husband, father. McCloskey had many decades to prepare himself for his transition from man to woman. His family had no such preparation. Only his mother accepted his decision with sympathy and understanding. McCloskey tells us that his sister, Laura, "was eleven years younger, a professor of psychology at the University of Arizona, a liberal woman with liberal views on gay rights and South Africa. Only later did Deirdre learn that her liberalism had limits."[5] When McCloskey informed her about his decision to cross, her instantaneous response was to diagnose him as mentally ill: "She decided, 'he's crazy,' the only reason her big brother would want to play at being her big sister."[6] It is odd that McCloskey, a libertarian, views liberals as tolerant.

McCloskey's prose is especially moving and effective in describing his sister's, his wife's, and his children's reactions to his self-disclosure. Oblivious to his inner turmoil and spiritual suffering, they cared only about the shame they felt that he was bringing on them. In an effort to placate them, McCloskey agreed to see a psychiatrist, thereby initiating a protracted and painful battle against the coalition of family members opposing his sex-change and their brutal psychiatric hatchet-men: "Donald's wife and sister were demanding that he be treated for 'mania.' Their notion was that he had gone crazy, and that if treated for the craziness he would drop the silliness about becoming a woman. *Maybe it would satisfy them.* The appointment was made for Donald's fifty-third birthday."[7]

It didn't satisfy them. It emboldened them. After a family conference, McCloskey's wife tells him: "'Last night I talked to your sister again. I'd like you to take pills for your mania. She wants to commit you as mentally incompetent.' / 'Jesus! How stupid can you get?' *He scorned the notion of a commitment.* She wanted him to be crazy. Treatably crazy."[8] Donald pleads with Laura: "I repeat: you shouldn't interfere.... You don't know me at all.... Be my sister, not my jailer." Laura is adamant: "But I love you."

On September 11, 1995, McCloskey goes to see a psychiatrist recommended by a colleague: *"That the crossers are free adults,* Deirdre reflected later, is not deemed pertinent. Another gender crosser put it so: 'When you want surgery on your nose, it's called a nose job. When you want surgery on your boobs, it's called a boob job. When you want surgery on your genitals...you're crazy!'"[9]

McCloskey rightly regards transsexual surgery as a type of cosmetic surgery. But the examples she cites serve her purpose poorly. A boob job enhances the person's chromosomal-social gender identity: it makes a woman more feminine looking. Transsexual surgery does the opposite: it transforms the person's chromosomal-social gender identity: it makes a male look like a female (or vice versa).[10] The remark, "When you want surgery on your genitals...you're crazy!" is too facile. A Christian male who converts to Judaism or Islam undergoes a circumcision, and psychiatrists do not call him crazy. It is easy to understand, however, that McCloskey was eager to minimize the intensity of the embarrassment his decision to cross was causing his sister, wife, and children.The psychiatrist in Iowa City concluded that McCloskey was transsexual and told him: "There is nothing I can do for you."[11] This time, Donald was lucky. But he was too naive about psychiatry. The doctor said, "There is nothing I can do *for you.*" He didn't say, "There is nothing another psychiatrist *might not be happy to do to you—for your sister.*" Donald tells his sister what happened. She becomes "furious.... 'I talked to your psychiatrist. He is an idiot,' she said emphatically." Donald protests: "Attempting to commit me was a stupid thing to do." He persists and Laura petitions to have him committed:

> He still didn't realize how close she had come.... He didn't know she was taking notes and writing down things like, "Irrationally angry.... I want my brother to be treated for his mania.... I love you. I want to help you."
>
> ... [S]omeone knocked hard on the door. The schnauzers barked hysterically as always, and his wife answered it. *Probably some delivery,* thought Dee [the name McCloskey uses between passing from Donald to Deirdre]. But he saw two uniformed men and got up. *What's this?* In came two sheriff's deputies in brown uniforms.
> "Sir, you have to come with us. We have a warrant."
> "A what!"
> "A warrant for arrest for mental examination."
> *"Good Lord, my sister's done it.".*..
> His sister and a former colleague of Dee's at the University of Chicago named David Galenson had used the civil commitment procedures designed to stop people from jumping off bridges.[12]

McCloskey was a "danger" to his sister: She was used to regarding him as her brother and was not about to change her mind about that.

> Dee offered no resistance to the sheriff's deputies and was cooperative. Libertarians like Dee appreciate that the core of state power is lethal violence. As a concession to his cooperative attitude and his social class, the deputies

agreed to cuff him with his hands in front instead of behind. Dee thought he was going to be given a chance to explain, and to show on the spot that he was not crazy. *The craziness is my sister's and Galenson's,* he thought. *Surely, this is all silliness, and a competent doctor will see immediately. Gender crossing is not illegal or evidence of craziness. I am going to have a nose job. There is no "danger to myself," that elastic cover for psychiatric thuggery. Surely, the psychiatrist will let me go home after this.*[13]

McCloskey was still optimistic. Or perhaps he was denying the reality of psychiatry, the kinds of sadisms of which the psychiatrists with whom he socialized were capable. McCloskey speaks of "psychiatric thuggery," but expects a non-thuggish psychiatrist to release him. Perhaps he didn't realize, or did not want to realize, that in America, *Anno Domini* 1995, the psychiatrist, too, is a captive—of his profession and the law.[14] As McCloskey discovered, there was no shortage of prominent psychiatrists, both at the University of Iowa and at the University of Chicago, happy to lock him up. "[T]he psychiatrists decided without telling him that they wanted him held for eight days. The feelings or condition or evidence or convenience or reputation of the victim are given no weight.... In Iowa, as in many states, any two people who claim to know the victim can have him committed for observation if they can lie successfully to a judge."[15]

As a rule, a little more than this is needed to pull off such a coup. As Erving Goffman observed, what is required is the construction of a "funnel of betrayal" by family members and friends.[16] In McCloskey's case, this is how the process unfolded. Mrs. McCloskey visits her husband in the psychiatric lockup. Counting on three decades of "love and marriage," he turns to her for help.

"Would you do me a favor?"

"What is it? I don't want to be involved." Dee resisted saying what he was thinking. *She does not want to be involved, she who could stop it at any time, saving me, as I certainly would save her. She could say: "This is ridiculous. This is my husband. He is perfectly sane. He is going to have a nose job. None of what his sister claims to have heard from me is true. Lay off!" The case against me would collapse.*[17]

Finally, McCloskey realizes his predicament, calls a lawyer, and gets himself a hearing before a judge.

Dee was indignant as his sister told her loving lies, and he kept passing notes to his lawyer. His sister testified on oath that her mother and brother had bi-polar affective disorder. "She is wrong," Dee scribbled. That her mother and brother had in fact been hospitalized for it. "That's not so."... On a speaker phone the district attorney interviewed David Galenson from the University of

Chicago.... Galenson's aged Aunt Eleanor, a retired psychoanalyst in New York was brought onto the speaker phone to testify. Dee sat dazed.... Then they did something that felt like torture. They called his son to testify.... Dee's son lived in far-off Chicago. Yet he testified, in words that sounded as if they were provided by the prosecutor herself, that to his own, nonhearsay knowledge his father was likely to flee if released on his own recognizance, a knowledge the son had no way of acquiring..... State-sponsored lying.... The competency hearing droned on into the afternoon. The judge complained that it was the longest he had experienced.[18]

McCloskey was released. But his sister wasn't finished. Two weeks after the commitment hearing in Iowa, McCloskey attends the annual meeting of the Social Science History Association at the Palmer House in Chicago, honoring him for his work on the rhetoric of economic history. A hotel employee hurries into the meeting room:

"Professor McCloskey, you are urgently needed outside. A phone call."

"What? What's happening?" As he got up: My God, my son here in Chicago has been hurt in a car accident. My wife is deathly ill. My daughter. He rushed out into the hallway.

And there was his sister, with two big Chicago policemen. Oh, my God, not again.

"I don't suppose you have informed the new judge that you've tried this once already in Iowa?"

Ignoring him, she ordered one of the policemen: "That's him. Seize him."[19]

McCloskey is incarcerated at the University of Chicago's teaching hospital. This time, he is duly alarmed: "[T]he doctor in charge, who in the evening settled the matter [that McCloskey was a proper subject for involuntary mental hospitalization], was a short, bossy man, unhappy with himself, Dee thought. He's never going to let any patient out, and he knows nothing of gender crossing." A woman psychiatrist, who McCloskey thought was sympathetic with his plight, came back to see him: "Dee said, 'I'm terrified of your colleague. Save me from him, please, please.' She didn't answer. The boss came back and declared that he was going to keep Dee. Maybe forever. With a show of taking care the doctor insisted that Dee ride up to the locked psychiatric ward in a wheelchair.... A creepy little man, Dee thought, dangerous, ignorant, a jailer."[20]

The battle over McCloskey's "mental health" was on in earnest, waged of course by lawyers, not doctors. It was war on a small scale but fought with great intensity, as wars between "loved ones" often are.

His sister had hired the second-best lawyer in the mental health bar of Chicago, using $10,000 she had lied to get out of their aged grandmother: "Donny's is sick, Granny. Mom won't help. You have to give me the money to help." Joel Mokyr, Jewish and a student of Irish history, was amused that this second-best lawyer was Jewish and that the first best, defending Dee was Irish. The two lawyers fought it out in a long hearing the day after Dee was seized... Dee's lawyer argued all afternoon with the judge, who finally in vexation threw the case into the hands of psychiatrists. You decide. But the doctors didn't want to decide.... *A month, a year. What does it matter? The patient has no right to freedom... They have every incentive,* Dee reflected, *to act as professional cowards.* Dee's lawyer worked and worked at hundreds of dollars an hour on the psychiatrist and finally persuaded him. *Probably out of fear of suit,* Dee imagined. *What if I were poor?*[21]

Laura McCloskey continued her efforts to secure "psychiatric treatment" for her brother. With the help of lawyers and tens of thousands of dollars in legal fees, McCloskey managed to escape another period of psychiatric imprisonment. Then, accepting a timely invitation to teach for a year in The Netherlands, he fled his sister, American psychiatry, and the United States. After returning to Iowa City, his wife divorced him:

She divorced, she would not meet, she moved to another town, she never shopped in Iowa City. No other contact. It was embarrassing. Mortifying.... Had Donald died of a heart attack at age fifty-three, as his father had, the wife would have acted the widow for a while, sad to see her life's companion leave, dignified in her grief. But, for God's sake, he became a woman.... Donald's wife would not speak or write, and Deirdre was inexperienced at a woman's imagination. *She feels that her marriage was meaningless. "Was I married all those years,"* she asks, *"to a woman? What does that make me?"*... Their son, a businessman in Chicago, late twenties, was also angry and ashamed.[22]

McCloskey's daughter also severed all relations with her father.

Transsexualism and Psychiatry

In *Crossing*, McCloskey does not identify his psychiatric jailers. However, in a personal communication, she has kindly told me the names of the psychiatrists responsible for diagnosing and detaining him as "dangerously mentally ill," and granted me permission to use that information. She wrote: "I have no objection whatever to you naming the names. None of them has ever expressed the slightest remorse about his or her behavior.... You can easily understand how my libertarian convictions about psychiatry were strengthened by the experience! I had your work in mind daily."[23]

In addition to the psychiatrists directly involved in McCloskey's commitment, Nancy Andreasen "had a tangential and in my opinion dishonorable role. I counted her a friend—we had known each other socially for many years. She...would not help when her colleagues grabbed me."[24] Andreasen—professor of psychiatry at the University of Iowa, editor-in-chief of the *American Journal of Psychiatry*, author, researcher, and recipient, in 2000, of a National Medal of Science Award—is one of the most famous and respected psychiatrists in America.

It is important to keep in mind that the psychiatric departments of the University of Iowa and University of Chicago medical schools are among the very "best" in the United States. The psychiatrists who incarcerated McCloskey are among the leaders of the psychiatric profession. They have the power to determine what counts as professionally correct psychiatric practice. They have the power to defame psychiatrists who limit their practice to treating only voluntary patients as irresponsible and dangerous quacks. They cannot be dismissed as ignoramuses practicing "psychiatric abuses" in some distant "unfree" country.

Because of my longstanding interest in both the medicalization of sex and the practice of involuntary mental hospitalization, I found *Crossings* doubly interesting and revealing. McCloskey's narrative illustrates many of the observations I have offered over the course of the past fifty years. In 1979, in an essay in the *New York Times Book Review*, I reminisced:

> When I was a medical student, if a man wanted to have his penis amputated, my psychiatric teachers said he suffered from schizophrenia, locked him up in an insane asylum, and threw away the key. Now, when I am a professor, my psychiatric colleagues say he is a "transsexual," my urological colleagues refashion his penis into a perineal cavity they call a "vagina," and *Time* magazine puts him on its cover and calls him "her." [I was referring to Richard/Renee Raskind.] Anyone who doubts that this is progress is considered to be ignorant of the discoveries of modern psychiatric sexology, a political reactionary, a sexual bigot, or something equally unflattering.[25]

I went on to suggest that the official definition of transsexualism as a disease "comes down to the strategic abuse of language," an effort to confuse and equate a biological phenomenon with a social role, chromosomal sexual identity with looking and acting like a woman/man. To clarify the debate about classifying the "condition," I raised the following hypothetical questions:

> Since "transsexualism" involves, is indeed virtually synonymous with, extensive surgical alterations of the normal human body, we might ask what

would happen, say, to a man who went to an orthopedic surgeon, told him that he felt like a right-handed person trapped in an ambidextrous body, and asked the doctor to cut off his perfectly healthy left arm? What would happen to a man who went to a urologist, told him that he felt like a Christian trapped in a Jewish body, and asked him to recover the glans of his penis with foreskin?[26]

I concluded that transsexualism is not a disease: "The transsexual male is indistinguishable from other males, save by his desire to be a woman.... If such a desire qualifies as a disease, transforming the desiring agent into a 'transsexual,' then the old person who wants to be young is a 'transchronological,' the poor person who wants to be rich is a 'transeconomical,' and so on." Clearly, psychiatrists do not classify all personal desires as diseases. The fact that they do so identify the desire for a change in sex roles is one of the manifestations of our living in a therapeutic state. Ostensibly, the "transsexers"—psychologists, psychiatrists, endocrinologists, urologists—are curing a disease; actually, they engage in the quasi-religious and political shaping and controlling of "masculine" and "feminine" behavior and identity.

The claim that males can be transformed, by means of hormones and surgery, into females, and vice versa, is a lie or a delusion. Chromosomal sex is fixed. And so are one's historical experiences of growing up and living as boy or girl, man or woman. What, then, can be achieved by means of so-called transsexual therapy? The language in which the reply is framed is crucial, and can never be neutral. Transsexual propagandists claim to transform "women trapped in men's bodies" into "real women." I claim that such persons are fake females, males who wear not only feminine clothing but also feminine-looking body parts.

In short, transsexual surgery is a type of cosmetic surgery, designed to make the body look "better" or "right," as those terms are understood by the subject electing to undergo the change. My insisting that transsexualism is not a disease does not mean that individuals who want to change their gender identity ought to be deprived of the liberty to do so. Aids to sexual crossings, like other personal services, ought to be sold and bought in the free market. Sadly, there is, in modern society, no legitimate space for thinking and speaking clearly about psychiatry. Even emphasizing the importance of differentiating between consensual psychiatric practices helping patients, and coercive psychiatric practices helping the patients' relatives but harming the patients, has become anathema.[27] The practices of psychiatric slavery are deeply embedded in our society. Even an account as fine as *Crossing*, written by so eminent a witness as Deirdre McCloskey, makes no impact on the unquestioning approval of this peculiar institution by bioethecists, journalists, and writers.

In his misguided and mistitled book, *Better Than Well*, Carl Elliott—who identifies himself as a bioethicist—writes at length about transsexuals and notes that many of them explain or rationalize their sex change by comparing it to a journey. His only comment about *Crossing* is: "'Gender crossing is a good deal like foreign travel,' writes Deirdre McCloskey, a transsexual economist."[28] Characteristically, the fact that psychiatrists twice incarcerated McCloskey is of no concern or interest to this "ethicist."

In a review of *Crossing* in the *New York Times*, the poet and writer Maxine Kumin praises the book as a fine piece of writing and naively attributes McCloskey's commitment to mistakes by poor psychiatrists:

> His sister and one of her academic colleagues played a sinister role in trying to thwart him. They conspired to have him committed as mentally incompetent—unfit to sign papers for optional surgical procedures.... Twice during his determined journey into womanhood, they managed to have him incarcerated—handcuffed, locked away where he could not harm himself, at first in the University of Iowa Hospital's mental ward and later in the University of Chicago Hospital—to await evaluations by psychiatrists whose knowledge of his situation was less than rudimentary.
>
> The shrinks he had the misfortune to encounter seemed still to be operating at a pre-60's level.[29]

The truth is that the psychiatrists McCloskey encountered were among the leaders of the profession, operating at a 1990s level. In Iowa, McCloskey's psychiatrists were Raymond Crowe, professor of psychiatry, an expert on genetics and developmental neurobiology, a "seasoned, well-funded researcher";[30] and Robert Robinson, professor and chairman of the Department of Psychiatry, a recognized researcher in neuropsychiatry, and former chairman of the Neurosciences Review Committee, National Institute of Mental Health. In Chicago, McCloskey's psychiatrist was Fred Ovsiew, a member of the American Psychoanalytic Association, associate professor of clinical psychiatry at the University of Chicago, and director of its Inpatient Psychiatric Unit.[31] These men cannot be dismissed the way Kumin dismisses them. The fact that she assumed the doctors who abused McCloskey were bungling psychiatric troglodytes speaks for itself.

Revealing her inability to see past the psychiatric rhetoric to the psychiatric slavery it conceals, Kumin remarks, "Gender crossers are still waiting for the gender identity disorder to be removed from the list of mental illnesses."[32] After their experiences with the mental health system, I would expect at least some gender crossers to scoff at psychiatric diagnoses and not care about what unpopular behaviors psychiatrists classify as diseases. During my own lifetime, psychiatrists have removed masturbation, fellatio, cunnilingus, and homosexuality from the list of mental illnesses, yet managed to triple and quadruple the number of disorders listed in the American Psychiatric Association's (APA) *Diagnostic and Statistical Manual*, adding, for example, caffeinism, nicotinism, dysmorphobia, and pathological gambling.

The legitimacy of psychiatry rests entirely on its being a branch of medicine. It has no legitimacy as a quasi-theological system allied with the state for the forcible resolving of family conflicts. Even if it were discovered that the feelings transsexuals experience are rooted in physicochemical processes in the body (in which case the phenomenon would be defined as an endocrinological disorder), the conflicts between the transsexual individual and the family members who oppose his or her decisions for sex change would remain.

Cosmetic surgery on a human being does not change the person's soul. Cosmetic surgery on the vocabulary of psychiatry does not change the profession's character.

Transsexualism in Perspective

By 2000, when *Crossing* was published, transsexualism had been widely discussed in the media for nearly thirty years. Jan (James) Morris's best-selling book, *Conundrum*—one of the earliest stories of a successful sex-change operation—was published in 1974. Born a man, Morris married, fathered five children before completing the sex transformation in 1972, and had a successful career as a journalist and writer, both as James and Jan. His wife accepted him as a woman without reservation.[33] Since then, numerous autobiographical and biographical accounts of sex-change operations and their personal consequences have been published.[34]

In 2001, the acclaimed director and playwright Jane Anderson wrote and produced a play, *Looking for Normal*. In 2003, retitled as *Normal*, she redid the story as a made-for-television film, featuring Tom Wilkinson and Jessica Lange as Roy and Irma Applewood, solid Midwesterners, a loving couple and devoted parents of two children. While celebrating their twenty-fifth wedding anniversary, Roy shocks Irma by confessing that he feels like a woman trapped in a man's body. "He wants an operation to make him the female he knows he is.... 'I want to go home,' is all Irma can say. But when she does find her voice, she has a question. 'When you're in bed, are you a man or a woman?' And when he insists he is going to have surgery, no matter whom it hurts, she declares, 'There's no way you're a woman. Only a man could be so selfish.'"[35] The marriage survives the sex-change operation.

The film earned high marks by critics. One reviewer commented: "Under Anderson's direction, surprise often gives way to a deeper understanding of a topic that, for many, remains incomprehensible.... 'I wanted to explore what makes a marriage last,' Anderson said. 'If you love somebody, what do you love? Do you love their body? Their gender? Their mind? Their heart? Their soul? And could someone be capable of loving another person who has gone through such a huge transformation?'"[36] These are the right questions to ask. These are the questions we ought to ask ourselves. However, we can do so *only if we are prepared to reject the psychiatrists' answers.*

McCloskey's account illustrates with dramatic clarity that psychiatrists do not ask questions about transsexualism. How could they? They already have a firm, "scientific" answer: "it" is a "disease." The psychiatrists' questions, if any, pertain only to "what kind of disease" does the "patient" have, what "causes" it, and how should the "disease be treated"? (This view may soon become politically incorrect. Psychiatrists will then change their minds, as they did with homosexuality, and claim to be ardent defenders and supporters of the rights of transsexuals.)

Neither Morris nor many others who chose sex-change surgery were committed as mad. Why, then, was McCloskey committed, not once but twice? I surmise because he had a sister who was a psychologist and a pious believer in mental illness as disease and psychiatric incarceration as treatment. She was in no way physically endangered by her brother's behavior. Nevertheless, she twice initiated psychiatric violence against him. *Cui bono?*

Laura McCloskey did not approve of her brother's decision to become a woman. She had no reason to approve of it. But neither had she any reason to commit him. She could have "divorced" him, that is, severed relations with him. In situations such as this, it is absurd for psychiatrists to "examine" the accused person for "evidence of mental illness." The conflict has more to do with the mental state of the accuser than it has with that of the accused.

The questions Anderson posed are the right ones. After a long marriage blessed by grown and healthy children, whom or what does each spouse love in the other? In the case of a wife, does she love her husband's body? His sexual services? His companionship? His soul? His money?

The lifestyle he provides? Could someone be capable of loving another person who has gone through a huge transformation? It is easier to see the problem McCloskey posed to his family if we detach it from sex, if we consider vast personal transformations that are not sexual in nature. I offer the following hypothetical case as an example.

You are happily married to a man for twenty-five years. He has had a successful career as an investment banker in Manhattan. You have made yourself a life appropriate to his income and social position, say, as a part-time book editor. On your twenty-fifth wedding anniversary, he tells you he is a medical missionary trapped in the life of an investment banker. He has followed a career in banking only because his father and grandfather were bankers and he did not want to disappoint them. Finally, he has decided to follow his heart. He will move to Nigeria and help dying AIDS patients. Would you accompany him? Wish him good luck and stay in Manhattan? Divorce him? Commit him?

Family problems of this type are far more common than most people are willing to acknowledge. The case of "Taliban John" is a real-life example. John Walker Lindh, baptized a Roman Catholic, grew up in Marin County, California. His father is a high-powered attorney. When John was fifteen, he read *The Autobiography of Malcolm X* and began to show an interest in the Muslim religion. After graduating from high school, he decided to become a Muslim and go to Yemen to study Arabic and memorize the Koran. One thing led to another and now he is "Taliban John," one of the most famous inmates in America's prison system. His parents not only approved his decision to convert to Islam and go to Yemen, they financed it. Had they, instead, decided that John might need psychiatric help, they could have taken him to a psychiatrist who might have concluded that he was showing early signs of schizophrenia and suggested commitment. The parents could then have committed John and perhaps saved him from the consequences of his choice.

Human ingenuity and modern technology, especially medical technology, make many kinds of behaviors and experiences available to us. The fact that a person can have a certain experience does not mean that it is good for him. Tolerating diverse sexual behaviors is not the same as accepting or approving them. There are many things to which we have a right that are not "right." Examples are hardly necessary.

Perhaps it should not surprise us that transsexualism is going the way of homosexuality, from serious mental illness justifying psychiatric incarceration to normal behavior and human right. In principle, this is good. In practice, in the therapeutic state in which we live, it is bad. Why?

Because any behavior recognized as "not pathological" is deemed, *ipso facto*, good or "valid," and taught to children in public schools.

The Spring 2003 issue of *City Journal* offers this report about Transgender, Bisexual, Gay, Lesbian Awareness Day ("To B GLAD Day") at a high school in Newton, Massachusetts:

> An advocacy session for students and teachers features three self-styled transgendered individuals—a member of the senior class and two recent graduates. One of the transgenders, born female, announces that "he" had been taking hormones for 16 months. "Right now I am a 14-year-old boy going through puberty and a 55-year-old woman going through menopause," she complains.... A second panelist declares herself an "androgyne in between both genders of society." She adds, "Gender is just a bunch of stereotypes from society, but I am completely personal, and my gender is fluid." Only in liberal Massachusetts could a public school endorse such an event for teens, you might think. But you would be wrong. For the last decade or so, largely working beneath public or parental notice, a well-organized movement has sought to revolutionize the curricula and culture of the nation's public schools. Its aim: to stamp out "hegemonic heterosexuality"—the traditional view that heterosexuality is the norm—in favor of a new ethos that does not just tolerate homosexuality but instead actively endorses experimenting with it, as well as with a polymorphous range of bisexuality, transgenderism, and transsexuality. The educational establishment has enthusiastically signed on.... This movement to "queer" the public schools, as activists put it, originated with a shift in the elite understanding of homosexuality.... There ensued a successful effort to normalize homosexuality throughout the culture, including a strong push for homosexual marriage, gays in the military, and other signs of civic equality. Underlying this militant stance was a radical new academic ideology called "queer theory."... Queer theory takes to its extreme limit the idea that all sexual difference and behavior is a product of social conditioning, not nature. It is, in their jargon, "socially constructed." For the queer theorist, all unambiguous and permanent notions of a natural sexual or gender identity are coercive impositions on our individual autonomy—our freedom to reinvent our sexual selves whenever we like.... A long list of well-known organizations has backed LGBT [Lesbian, Gay, Bisexual, Transgender] programs in the classroom, including the American Psychiatric Association, the American Library Association, and the National Association of Social Workers. No organization has been more steadfast in its support of GLSEN [Gay, Lesbian and Straight Educational Network] than the NEA [National Education Association].[37]

So, why was McCloskey twice committed to a mental hospital? Because his sister preferred to think of him as mentally ill rather than as a person who made a difficult and momentous decision, and because psychiatrists are in the business of locking up people. As Anton Pavlovich

Chekhov (1860-1904) memorably put it: "Since prisons and madhouses exist, why, somebody is bound to sit in them. If not you, then I; if not I, then some third person."[38]

Role Obligation and Psychiatric Coercion

Laura McCloskey's conviction that her brother was "crazy" and had to be "treated" for a "mental illness," whether he liked it or not, displays dramatically the "political" character of the process of psychiatric commitment. At the same time, it demonstrates that the process has not the remotest resemblance to the diagnosis and treatment of disease, with the consent of the patient.

From the point of view of scientific medicine, disease is a physical-chemical derangement of the human body. Because the body belongs to its owner, the so-called patient, the physician can have access to it—can diagnose and treat it—only with the consent of the patient.

The pain McCloskey was causing his family, especially his sister, did not originate in his body. It originated in his relationship with them, specifically, in what they viewed as his failure to fulfill his role obligation to them.

I began this chapter by observing that our most basic, albeit involuntary, "contract" with our fellow man is our chromosomally determined—and, later, socially and legally defined—sexual identity. I now want to expand briefly on this important point.

In the modern world, we are accustomed to thinking of an obligation as a duty we incur because we voluntarily assume it, exemplified by an explicit agreement or contract. However, this is only a small part of the sum total of our obligations.

We, moderns, view ourselves as individuals. It was not always thus. The idea of the individual is, in part, an existential fiction. There has never been and there never can be a human being in isolation from other human beings. *We exist only in relation to others.*[39] In the premodern world and in tribal societies today, social relations are regulated by status, that is, by the obligations that adhere to the person's role in the family and society. In Sir Henry Maine's classic formulation, "... we may say that the movement of the progressive societies has hitherto been a movement *from Status to Contract."*[40]

It is obvious, however, that cooperation among individuals cannot rest solely on legally enforceable contracts, that there must be a large area of human affairs regulated by obligations adhering to roles. Some roles we assume voluntarily, for example, husband and wife, doctor, teacher, and so forth; and we are then expected—by a combination of custom, law, morality, and what is best called "role obligation"—to fulfill our role, be loyal or true to it.[41]

In addition to roles we assume voluntarily, there are others that are ascribed or assigned to us, exemplified by the role of the child. No child asks to be born. Nor does he ask to be male or female, Christian or Jew, American or Hungarian. These and many other roles and statuses are assigned to the child and he is then expected to fulfill the attached obligations. The importance of this type of expectation is revealed by the rich vocabulary we have to describe the correct fulfillment of a role obligation, such as dependability, reliability, faithfulness, fidelity, piety, loyalty, devotion, and trustworthiness.

The true source of McCloskey's predicament was his "unfaithfulness" to his role as male, as son, brother, husband, and father. It had nothing to do with illness and medicine. In principle, rejection of one's gender role resembles rejection of one's role as a member of a religious community or as a citizen of a particular country. We might note in this connection that there is a custom in some Orthodox Jewish circles that, if a child intermarries, the child's family is expected to sit *shiva* (that is, mourn) for him as if he had died and then shun him.

In McCloskey's case, different members of his family reacted differently to his desire to "convert" from male to female. His mother accepted it. His wife and children did not and shunned him. His sister defined it as a symptom of "mental illness and dangerousness to self" and successfully initiated psychiatric violence against him.

Conclusions

For centuries, psychiatrists regarded socially unacceptable forms of sexual behavior as the symptoms of serious mental diseases. They still do. The psychiatrist's role as agent of social control has not changed. Social conventions regarding sexual behavior have.[42]

In 2000, the APA and the *DSM* replaced the term "transsexualism" with the term "gender identity disorder." What is Gender Identity Disorder? It is transsexualism. *DSM-IV* offers a three-page description of its "diagnostic features" and then states: "There is no diagnostic test specific for Gender Identity Disorder."[43] No matter. It's a real disease: "Despite intensive biological and psychological research, the aetiology of the gender identity disorder remains an enigma. It may well be an interaction of genetic, hormonal and subtle psychodynamic factors awaiting elucidation. In the meantime, consistent, careful and informed classification is of paramount importance to diagnosis and treatment."[44]

Kaplan & Sadock's Synopsis of Psychiatry, one of the most frequently used psychiatric texts in medical schools and psychiatric residency programs, states: "Transsexualism: The individual desires to live and be accepted as a member of the opposite sex, usually accompanied by the wish to make his body as congruent as possible with the preferred sex through surgery and hormonal treatment.[45]

The psychiatric perspective on transsexualism pits the psychiatrist against the patient, and vice versa. The psychiatrist views the subject as a lunatic troublemaker, and himself as a scientist and healer whose professional duty is to diagnose the patient "correctly" and treat him "appropriately." The patient does not view himself as ill and is not interested in being diagnosed. However, he needs the psychiatrist to provide him with goods and services that, in our society, only physicians licensed to practice medicine can provide legally; specifically, he needs the psychiatrist to certify him as "mentally fit" to receive the drugs and surgery necessary for the sex change.

Gender is not the only marker of our personal identity ascribed to us by biology or society. Age, religion, nationality, and native tongue are some others. Using transsexualism as a model, we could, as I noted earlier, construct many other kinds of "Personal Identity Disorders," such as the following:

- Transdenominationalism: The individual wants to live and be accepted as a member of the "opposite" religion (for example, Christian as Muslim), accompanied by the desire to make his body conform to the requirements of the preferred creed through reconstructive surgery (circumcision).

- Transnationalism, usually a dual diagnosis disorder, accompanied by Translingualism: The individual wants to live and be accepted as a member of the "opposite" nationality (for example, Hungarian as American), accompanied by the desire to make his place of residence as congruent as possible with his preferred nationality, through emigration and by learning a new language.

- Transchronologicalism: The individual wants to live and be accepted as a member of a younger age group than his chronological peer group, typically accompanied by the desire to make his appearance and body as congruent as possible with the preferred age group through dress, makeup, and plastic surgery.

The list could be expanded by adding identity "crossings" affecting a role that the person has assumed voluntarily but wishes to exchange for another, for example, occupation or marital status:

- Transoccupationalism: The individual wants to live and be accepted as a member of an occupation more lucrative and prestigious than his own, typically accompanied by the desire to make his credentials and persona as congruent as possible with the those possessed by the mimicked profession, by earning or faking the credentials required for membership in the new occupation.[46]

- Transmaritalism: The individual wants to live and be accepted as a member of a marital state more comfortable than the one in which he finds himself, typically accompanied by the desire to be married if he is single, and be divorced if he is married, by taking the actions necessary to achieve his aim.

The point is that physicians possess socially authenticated authority to define what counts as a "disease." Psychiatrists possess legally legitimized power to define what counts as a "mental disorder," what counts as "dangerousness to self or others," and to incarcerate individuals so diagnosed. This is the lesson the psychiatric profession's crime against McCloskey teaches us.

Finale

Libertarians view the state as an organization that possesses a monopoly on the legitimate use of coercion. This does not mean that libertarians do not recognize that, *inter alia*, the state may also deliver certain services, such as postal services, railroad services, and health care services. It means only that they consider the state's monopoly over the legitimate use of coercion its most distinctive and most important feature.

Because the inmates of so-called "mental hospitals" are and have always been incarcerated, it has always seemed to me obvious that psychiatry is an arm of the coercive apparatus of the state. The justifications for psychiatrists' possessing a monopoly on the legitimate use of medical coercion are psychiatric, therapeutic, and criminologic: mental illness, the mental patient's lack of insight into his illness and need for treatment, and the patient's and public's need for protection from dangerousness due to mental illness. This does not mean that I do not recognize that, *inter alia*, psychiatrists may also deliver certain services that people want and of which they voluntarily avail themselves. It means only that I consider the psychiatric profession's monopoly on the legitimate use of coercion its most distinctive and most important feature.

Everyone knows that the state possesses power to force people to do what they do not want to do, and to forcibly prevent them from doing what they want to do. George Washington, the *primus inter pares* of the Founding Fathers, warned: "Government is not reason; it is not eloquence; it is force."[1] Against the dangers represented by the state as an apparatus of coercion, we have a measure of protection in the Bill of Rights and the rule of law.

However, few people know, and even fewer admit, that the modern state also possesses a very different kind of power, namely, the power to forcibly diagnose persons as mentally ill and treat their alleged mental illness against their will; that is, to stigmatize innocent individuals as insane and deprive them of liberty by incarcerating them in prisons called hospitals. Against the dangers represented by the state as an apparatus of "therapy," we have no formal, legally enforceable protection. The differences between these two dangers to liberty and responsibility may be illustrated as follows.

- The welfare state seeks to *relieve poverty and unemployment*; its beneficiaries are not helped against their will; it is a constitutional state, regulated by the rule of law. The recipient of a welfare check who gives the money to a friend or uses it to buy liquor is not persecuted and punished by agents of the welfare state.

- The therapeutic state seeks to *remedy personal and social problems defined as diseases*; its beneficiaries are often "helped" against their will; it is a totalitarian state, governed by the rule of therapeutic discretion. The recipient of psychiatric medication who gives the drug to a friend or refuses to avail himself of its "benefits" is persecuted and punished by agents of the therapeutic state.

As I stated in the Preface, the principles and practices of deinstitutionalization, outpatient commitment, the mental patient's right to treatment, and the psychiatrist's duty to protect have effectively erased the line between the legal statuses of voluntary and involuntary, confined and unconfined patients; transformed all mental patients into persons actually or potentially not responsible for their actions, hence subject to psychiatric coercions; and rendered all mental health professionals responsible for their patients' misbehavior and welfare, with the duty to coerce them if necessary. This is why I hold that noncoercive psychiatry is an oxymoron.

It is easier to see a moral evil and political wrong than to correct it. The abomination of slavery was evident to many Americans before the United States was born in 1776. A century and a bloody war later, its abolition was still more fiction than fact.

In contrast, most Americans view psychiatric slavery not as evil, but as good. This is likely to remain the case so long as most people believe the "scientific" fables of psychiatrists with the same reverence and lack of critical judgment with which they believed, and often still believe, the religious fables of priests. At one time, organized American religion, law, and medicine supported chattel slavery, that is, the alliance of slavery and the state. Now, they support psychiatric slavery, the alliance of psychiatry and the state. Abolishing this abomination is an idea whose time has, assuredly, not (yet) come.

Acknowledgments

I am, once again, deeply indebted to my family, friends, colleagues, and fans for conversations, criticisms, suggestions, and sources; for reading and correcting the manuscript; and, last but not least, for considering my views, widely regarded as wrongheaded or worse, valid and worthy of support.

My brother George continued unfailingly to give me the benefit of his wide knowledge and good judgment, and Peter Uva, librarian at the SUNY Upstate Medical University, his unstintingly generous help supplying the reference materials I needed for this book.

My daughter Margot and son-in-law Steve Peters, and Walter Block, Nicolas Martin, Jeffrey Schaler, Mira de Vries, and Roger Yanow critiqued the entire manuscript (sometimes more than once). Deirdre McCloskey provided information and permission to publish details about her personal encounters with psychiatrists. Chris Matthew Sciabarra gave invaluable help with the chapter on Ayn Rand. Michael Paley, my editor at Transaction Publishers, offered a steady stream of valuable advice, saved me from blunders, and did a fine job of editing the manuscript.

I thank all of them, and others not mentioned, for their interest, good will, and support.

I also thank Professor Deirdre N. McCloskey and the University of Chicago Press for permission to reprint material from *Crossing: A Memoir* (Chicago: University of Chicago Press, 1999), © by The University of Chicago. All rights reserved. Published 1999.

Notes

Epigraph

1. Friedrich von Hayek, *The Constitution of Liberty* (Chicago: University of Chicago Press, 1960), p. 31.

Preface

1. Thomas Szasz, "Commitment of the mentally ill: Treatment or social restraint?" *Journal of Nervous and Mental Disease*, 125: 293-307 (April-June), 1957; *The Myth of Mental Illness: Foundations of a Theory of Personal Conduct* [1961], revised edition (New York: HarperCollins, 1974); *Psychiatric Slavery: When Confinement and Coercion Masquerade as Cure* [1977] (Syracuse: Syracuse University Press, 1998); *Insanity: The Idea and Its Consequences* [1987] (Syracuse: Syracuse University Press, 1997); *Liberation By Oppression: A Comparative Study of Slavery and Psychiatry* (New Brunswick, NJ: Transaction Publishers, 2002).

2. John Stuart Mill, *The Subjection of Women* [1869] (Cambridge: MIT Press, 1970), pp. 1, 5.

3. Thomas Szasz, *Liberation By Oppression*, op. cit.

4. See especially Thomas Szasz, *The Manufacture of Madness: A Comparative Study of the Inquisition and the Mental Health Movement* [1970] (Syracuse: Syracuse University Press, 1997).

5. See Thomas Szasz, *Pharmacracy: Medicine and Politics in America* [2001] (Syracuse: Syracuse University Press, 2003).

6. Henry Sumner Maine, *Ancient Law: Its Connection with the Early History of Society, and Its Relation to Modern Ideas* [1864], Foreword by Lawrence Rosen (Tucson: University of Arizona Press, 1986), p. 165, emphasis in the original.

7. Marcia Goin, "From the president. The 'suicide-prevention contract': A dangerous myth," *Psychiatric News*, 38: 3, 27 (July 18), 2003. http://pn.psychiatryonline.org/cgi/content/full/38/14/3

8. Daniel Luchins, "Mental illness, rights" (book review), *JAMA*, 290: 674-675 (August 6), 2003, p. 475.

9. James C. Beck, editor, *Confidentiality Versus the Duty to Protect: Foreseeable Harm in the Practice of Psychiatry* (Washington, DC: American Psychiatric Press, 1990); Gary A. Chaimowitz, Graham D. Glancy, and Janice Blackburn, "The duty to warn and protect: Impact on practice," *Canadian Journal of Psychiatry*, 45: 899-904, 2000.

10. For discussion and documentation, see Thomas Szasz, "Noncoercive psychiatry: An oxymoron," *Journal of Humanistic Psychology*, 31: 117-125 (Spring), 1991; *Fatal Freedom: The Ethics and Politics of Suicide* [1999] (Syracuse: Syracuse University Press, 2002); *Pharmacracy*, op. cit.; and *Liberation By Oppression*, op. cit.

11. See for example, Benno Mueller-Hill, "The blood from Auschwitz and the silence of the scholars," *History and Philosophy of the Life Sciences*, 21: 331-365, 1999.

12.   Dante Alighieri, *The Inferno*, translated by John Ciardi (New York: Mentor, 1954), pp. 42-43. Dante scholar John D. Sinclair calls these sinners "neutrals" and considers them guilty of the vice of cowardice. Dante Alighieri, *The Divine Comedy of Dante Alighieri*, translated by John D. Sinclair (New York: Oxford University Press, 1968), pp. 54-55.

13.   For information regarding the Austrian School of Economics (briefly, Austrian Economics), see Edwin Dolan, editor, *The Foundations of Modern Austrian Economics* (Kansas City: Sheed and Ward, 1976) and Richard M. Ebeling, *Austrian Economics and the Political Economy of Freedom* (Northhampton, MA: Edward Elgar, 2003); also, Hansjoerg Klausinger, "From Mises to Morgenstern: The Austrian School of Economics during the Standestaat," no date, http://www.mises.org/journals/scholar/Klausinger.pdf

14.   See Richard Yeo, *Defining Science: William Whewell, Natural Knowledge, and Public Debate in Early Victorian England* (Cambridge: Cambridge University Press, 1993), especially pp. 231-237; "William Whewell," *Stanford Encyclopedia of Philosophy*. http://plato.stanford.edu/entries/whewell; see also Eugene P. Wigner, "The Unreasonable Effectiveness of Mathematics in the Natural Sciences," in Timothy Ferris, editor, *The World Treasury of Physics, Astronomy, and Mathematics* (Boston: Little, Brown and Company, 1991), pp. 526-540.

15.   Michael Polanyi, "Life's Irreducible Structures" [1968], in Michael Polanyi, *Knowing and Being*, edited by Marjorie Greene (Chicago: University of Chicago Press, 1968), p. 238; see generally, Michael Polanyi, *Personal Knowledge: Towards a Post-Critical Philosophy* (Chicago: University of Chicago Press, 1958) and *Science, Faith, and Society* (Chicago: Phoenix Books/University of Chicago Press, 1964).

Introduction

1.   John Crammer, "1941-1950," in Hugh Freeman, editor, *A Century of Psychiatry* (London: Mosby-Wolfe/Harcourt Publishers, 1999), p. 146, emphasis added.

2.   John Crammer, *Asylum History: Buckinghamshire County Pauper Lunatic Asylum—St. John's* (London: Gaskell, 1990), p. x.

3.   See Thomas Szasz, *Law, Liberty, and Psychiatry: An Inquiry into the Social Uses of Psychiatry* [1963] (Syracuse: Syracuse University Press, 1989); and *Psychiatric Justice* [1965] (Syracuse: Syracuse University Press, 1988).

4.   SpicyQuotes.com. http://www.theuseful.com/p_pitch.htm?record_promo_id=894

5.   Mary L. Durham, "Civil Commitment of the Mentally Ill: Research, Policy, and Practice," in Bruce D. Sales and Saleem A. Shah, editors, *Mental Health and Law: Research, Policy, and Services* (Durham, N.C.: Carolina Academic Press, 1996), pp. 17-40; p. 17.

6.   Robert M. Levy and Leonard S. Rubenstein, *The Rights of People with Mental Disabilities: The Authoritative ACLU Guide to the Rights of People with Mental Illness and Mental Retardation* (Carbondale, IL: Southern Illinois University Press, 1996), p. 302.

7.   Thomas Szasz, *Liberation By Oppression: A Comparative Study of Slavery and Psychiatry* (New Brunswick, NJ: Transaction Publishers, 2002).

8.   John E.E.D Acton, *Selected Writings of Lord Acton: Essays in the Study and Writing of History,* edited by J. Rufus Fears, 3 vols. (Indianapolis: Liberty Classics, 1988), vol. 3, pp. 491, 490.

9.   Gilbert K. Chesterton, *Orthodoxy* (London: John Lane, 1909), p. 32.

10. Edmund Burke, *Reflections on the Revolution in France* [1790], Foreword by Francis Canavan (Indianapolis: Liberty Fund, 1999), pp. 94, 93.

11. John E.E.D. Acton, *Selected Writings of Lord Acton*, op. cit., vol. 3, p. 495.

12. Benito Mussolini, quoted in Michael J. Oakeshott, *The Doctrine of Fascism*, by Benito Mussolini, in *The Social and Political Doctrines of Contemporary Europe* (Cambridge: Cambridge University Press, 1939). Cited from: http: www.constitution.org/tyr/mussolini.htm

13. Jacob L. Talmon, *The Origin of Totalitarian Democracy* (New York: Frederick A. Praeger, 1960); Thomas Szasz, *Pharmacracy: Medicine and Politics in America* [2001] (Syracuse: Syracuse University Press, 2003).

14. Roger Scruton, "The political problem of Islam," *Intercollegiate Review*, 38: 3-15 (Fall), 2002, pp. 5, 9.

15. G. Brock Chisholm, "The psychiatry of enduring peace and social progress," *Psychiatry*, 9: 3-9, 1946; p. 9; and G. Brock Chisholm, quoted in, Daniel Callahan, "The WHO Definition of Health," in, Rem B. Edwards and Glenn C. Garber, editors, *Bio-Ethics* (New York: Harcourt Brace Jovanovich, 1988), pp. 257-266; pp. 259-260.

16. Thomas Szasz, *Pharmacracy*, op. cit.

17. Albert Camus, *The Rebel: An Essay on Man in Revolt* [1951], translated by Anthony Bower (New York: Vintage Books, 1956), p. 4.

18. See chapter 10.

19. Institute for Justice. http://www.ij.org. http://www.ij.org/index.shtml

20. The Cato Institute. http://www.cato.org/about/about.html

21. Official web site of the Libertarian Party, www.lp.org.

22. National Platform of the Libertarian Party. Adopted in Convention, July 2002, Indianapolis, Indiana. http://www.lp.org/issues/platform/platform_all.html

23. James Madison, "Letter to William Bradford," April 1, 1774, quoted in James Samples, "James Madison's vision of liberty," *CATO Policy Report*, 23: 1 and 10-12 (March/April), 2001, p. 12.

24. Albert Camus, "The Wager of Our Civilization" [1957], in *Resistance, Rebellion, and Death*, translated by Justin O'Brien (New York: Knopf, 1961), p. 240.

25. Francis Fukuyama," The fall of the libertarians: Sept. 11 might have also brought down a political movement," *OpinionJournal*, September 12, 2003. http://opinionjournal.com/editorial/feature.html?id=105002013

26. Edmund Burke, "A letter from Mr. Burke to a Member of the National Assembly in answer to some objections to his book on French Affairs" [1791], in Edmund Burke, *The Works of the Right Honorable Edmund Burke*, 12 vols. (Boston: Wells & Lilly, 1826), vol. 3, p. 315.

27. John E.E.D. Acton, *Selected Writings of Lord Acton*, op. cit., 490.

28. Thomas Szasz, *Ideology and Insanity: Essays on the Psychiatric Dehumanization of Man* [1970] (Syracuse: Syracuse University Press, 1991).

29. Thomas Szasz, *Law, Liberty, and Psychiatry*, op. cit.; *The Manufacture of Madness: A Comparative Study of the Inquisition and the Mental Health Movement* [1970] (Syracuse: Syracuse University Press, 1997); *Insanity: The Idea and Its Consequences* [1987] (Syracuse: Syracuse University Press, 1997); *Cruel Compassion: The Psychiatric Control of Society's Unwanted* [1994] (Syracuse: Syracuse University Press, 1998); *Pharmacracy*, op. cit.; and *Liberation By Oppression*, op. cit.

30. Lawrence Kootnikoff, "Victim's kin can sue psychiatrists," *Los Angeles Daily Journal*, August 19, 2003, p. 2.

31.   Leonie Lamont and Miguel Holland, "Judge awards woman's insane killer $300,000," *Sydney Morning Herald* (Australia), August 20, 2003. http://www.smh.com.au/articles/2003/08/19/1061261156746.html
32.   Thomas Szasz, *Liberation By Oppression*, op. cit.; see also, Thomas Szasz, *Cruel Compassion*, op. cit.

Chapter 1. Responsibility

1.   Thomas Szasz, *A Lexicon of Lunacy: Metaphoric Malady, Personal Responsibility, and Psychiatry* (New Brunswick, NJ: Transaction Publishers, 1993).
2.   Thomas Szasz, *Insanity: The Idea and Its Consequences* [1987] (Syracuse: Syracuse University Press, 1997); "Psychiatry and the control of dangerousness: On the apotropaic function of the term 'mental illness,'" *Journal of Medical Ethics*, 29: 227-230 (August), 2003.
3.   James Madison, "Property," in *The Writings of James Madison*, edited by Gaillard Hunt, 9 vols. (New York: G. P. Putnam's Sons, 1900-1910), vol. 6, p. 103.
4.   Garet Garrett, "The people's pottage," quoted in *Freedom Daily*, 4: 29-32 (July), 1933, p. 32.
5.   See Thomas Szasz, *Insanity*, op. cit.; *Ceremonial Chemistry: The Ritual Persecution of Drugs, Addicts, and Pushers* [1976] (Syracuse: Syracuse University Press, 2003); *Our Right to Drugs: The Case for a Free Market* [1992] (Syracuse: Syracuse University Press, 1996); and *Fatal Freedom: The Ethics and Politics of Suicide* [1999] (Syracuse: Syracuse University Press, 2002).
6.   Adam Smith, quoted in Edwin G. West, *Adam Smith: The Man and His Works* (Indianapolis: Liberty Press, 1976), p. 16.
7.   Bruce Ramsay, "Dialog with an absolutist," *Liberty*, 17: 29-30, 53 (July), 2003.
8.   Thomas Szasz, *Pharmacracy: Medicine and Politics in America* [2001] (Syracuse: Syracuse University Press, 2003); *Liberation By Oppression: A Comparative Study of Slavery and Psychiatry* (New Brunswick, NJ: Transaction Publishers, 2002).
9.   Thomas Szasz, "Involuntary mental hospitalization: A crime against humanity," *Exchange*, December, 1967, pp. 1-4; "The crime of commitment," *Psychology Today*, 2: 55-57 (March), 1969.
10.   Llewellyn H. Rockwell, Jr., "Freedom is Not 'Public Policy,'" June 17, 2002, http://www.mises.org/fullstory.asp?control=979, emphasis added.
11.   Friedrich A. Hayek, *The Fatal Conceit: The Errors of Socialism,* edited by W. W. Bartley, III (Chicago: University of Chicago Press, 1989).

Chapter 2. The Libertarian Credo and the Ideology of Psychiatry

1.   http://www.4literature.net/Henry_David_Thoreau/Civil_Disobedience/
2.   "The Jeffersonian perspective." http://www.geocities.com/CapitolHill/ 7970/jefpco09.htm
3.   Francis Hutcheson, *Inquiry into the Origins of our Ideas of Beauty and Virtue, in Two Treatises* (1725). http://www.ask.co.uk/
4.   "Utilitarianism." http://sol.brunel.ac.uk/~jarvis/bola/ethics/utility.html
5.   http://www.spartacus.schoolnet.co.uk/PRbentham.htm; Davis Hume, *Hume's Ethical Writings: Selections from David Hume,* edited and with an Introduction by Alasdair MacIntyre (Notre Dame, IN: University of Notre Dame Press, 1965).
6.   John Stuart Mill, *Utilitarianism* [1863], in *Essential Works of John Stuart Mill,* edited by Max Lerner (New York: Bantam Books, 1961).

7. John E.E.D. Acton, *Selected Writings of Lord Acton: Essays in the Study and Writing of History,* edited by J. Rufus Fears, 3 vols. (Indianapolis: Liberty Classics, 1988), vol. 3, pp. 490-491.

8. Dean Russell, "What is a libertarian?" http://www.libertarians.net/lib-lp-s.html; http://www.boogieonline.com/revolution/politics/name.html

9. John Locke, *The Second Treatise of Government,* in *Two Treatises of Government* [1690], edited by Peter Laslett (New York: New American Library, 1965), p. 350, emphasis added.

10. Murray N. Rothbard, *For a New Liberty: The Libertarian Manifesto,* revised edition (New York: Collier Macmillan, 1978), p. 23.

11. Walter Block, "Jonah Goldberg and the libertarian axiom on non-aggression," June 28, 2001. http://www.lewrockwell.com/orig/block1.html

12. Murray N. Rothbard, *For a New Liberty,* op. cit., p. 90.

13. Official web site of the Libertarian Party, www.lp.org, and National Platform of the Libertarian Party, Adopted in Convention, July 2002, Indianapolis, Indiana. http://www.lp.org/issues/platform/platform_all.html

14. Edmund A. Opitz, *The Libertarian Theology of Freedom* (Tampa, FL: Hallberg Publishing Corporation, 1999).

15. "Charles Murray—Libertarian," http://www.self-gov.org/murray.html.

16. Charles Murray, *What It Means to Be a Libertarian: A Personal Interpretation* (New York: Broadway Books, 1997).

17. H. C. Black, *Black's Law Dictionary,* revised 4th edition (St. Paul: West, 1968), p. 890.

18. Thomas Szasz, *The Myth of Mental Illness: Foundations of a Theory of Personal Conduct* [1961], revised edition (New York: HarperCollins, 1974).

19. Quoted in Robert Higgs, *Crisis and Leviathan: Critical Episodes in the Growth of American Government* (New York: Oxford University Press, 1987), p. 159.

20. G. J. Danton, quoted in *Bartlett's Familiar Quotations,* edited by Justin Kaplan, 16th ed., p. 364.

21. This volume, chapter 3.

22. See Thomas Szasz, *Schizophrenia: The Sacred Symbol of Psychiatry* [1976] (Syracuse: Syracuse University Press, 1988) and *The Meaning of Mind: Language, Morality, and Neuroscience* [1996] (Syracuse: Syracuse University Press, 2002).

23. David Bergland, *Libertarianism in One Lesson* (Costa Mesa, CA: Orpheus Publications, 1984), p. 5.

24. Gilbert K. Chesterton, *Orthodoxy* (London: John Lane, 1909), p. 32. See also, http://www.the700club.org/bibleresources/theology/chesterton.

25. Edmund A. Opitz, *The Libertarian Theology of Freedom* (Tampa, FL: Hallberg Publishing Corporation, 1999), p. 26.

26. H. L. Mencken, quoted in ibid., pp. 64-65.

27. Edmund A. Opitz, *The Libertarian Theology of Freedom,* op. cit., p. 65, emphasis added.

28. Charles Hallberg, "Foreword," in Edmund A. Opitz, *The Libertarian Theology of Freedom,* op. cit, pp. 9-10; p. 9.

29. *Union Pacific Railway Co. v. Botsford,* 141 U.S. 250, 251 (1891).

30. *Olmstead v. United States,* 277 U.S. 438 (1928), p. 479.

31. *Application of President and Directors of Georgetown College,* 331 F. 2nd, 1010 (D.C. Cir. 1964); emphasis in the original.

32. *Thor v. Superior Court (Andrews),* 855 P.2d 375 (Cal. 1993); pp. 375, 376, 384. The court was citing *In re Osborne* (D.C. 1972) 294 A. 2d 372, 375, fn. 5.

33.   See Thomas Szasz, *Insanity: The Idea and Its Consequences* [1987] (Syracuse: Syracuse University Press, 1997), Thomas Szasz, *Pharmacracy: Medicine and Politics in America* [2001] (Syracuse: Syracuse University Press, 2003), and *Liberation By Oppression: A Comparative Study of Slavery and Psychiatry* (New Brunswick, NJ: Transaction Publishers, 2002).

34.   http://quotes.prolix.nu/Authors/?Goethe

Chapter 3. Economics and Psychiatry

1.   See Michael D. Aeschliman, *The Restitution of Man: C. S. Lewis and the Case Against Scientism* (Grand Rapids, MI: Eerdmans Publishing Company, 1998); also Hayek's critique of scientism in his Nobel Banquet Lecture, this volume, chapter 4.

2.   For further details, see Thomas Szasz, *Cruel Compassion: The Psychiatric Control of Society's Unwanted* [1994] (Syracuse: Syracuse University Press, 1998), especially chapter 7, "Economics and Psychiatry."

3.   Robert H. Nelson, *Economics as Religion: From Samuelson to Chicago and Beyond* (University Park: Pennsylvania State University Press, 2001).

4.   Ibid., pp. xv, xx-xxi; see also Robert H. Nelson, *Reaching for Heaven on Earth: The Theological Meaning of Economics* (Lanham, MD: Rowman and Littlefield, 1991).

5.   Thomas Szasz, *The Myth of Psychotherapy: Mental Healing as Religion, Rhetoric, and Repression* [1978] (Syracuse: Syracuse University Press, 1988).

6.   Robert H. Nelson, *Economics as Religion*, op. cit., pp. 300, 17.

7.   John Maynard Keynes, *The General Theory of Employment, Interest, and Money* (New York: Harcourt, Brace, 1936), p. 298.

8.   Norbert Wiener, *God and Golem, Inc.: A Comment on Certain Points where Cybernetics Impinges on Religion* (Cambridge: M.I.T. Press, 1964), pp. 88-91, emphasis added.

9.   This volume, chapter 4.

10.   Robert Higgs, "Know thy enemy," *Reason*, 25: 38 (December), 1993, emphasis added.

11.   Thomas Szasz, *Ceremonial Chemistry: The Ritual Persecution of Drugs, Addicts, and Pushers* [1976] (Syracuse: Syracuse University Press, 2003).

12.   Wilhelm Röpke, *A Humane Economy: The Special Framework of the Free Market* (Indianapolis: Liberty Fund, 1971), pp. 248-249.

13.   Donald (Deirdre) N. McCloskey, *The Rhetoric of Economics* (Madison: University of Wisconsin Press, 1985).

14.   Donald (Deirdre) N. McCloskey, "The rhetoric of economic development," *The Cato Journal*, 7: 249-254 (Spring/Summer), 1987; p. 249.

15.   Donald (Deirdre) N. McCloskey, *The Rhetoric of Economics*, op. cit., p. 3.

16.   Peter Bauer, "The disregard of reality," *The Cato Journal*, 7:29-42 (Spring/Summer), 1987, p. 33.

17.   Wilhelm Röpke, *A Humane Economy*, op. cit., p. 247.

18.   Ibid., p. 15.

19.   Ibid., p. 16.

20.   Ibid., pp. 62, 138, 185.

21.   Ludwig von Mises, *Human Action: A Treatise on Economics* (New Haven: Yale University Press, 1949), p. 92. For more about Mises, see this volume, chapter 10.

22. Friedrich von Wieser, *Social Economics* [1914], translated by A. Ford Hinrichs (New York: Greenberg, 1927), p. 3. See generally Richard M. Ebeling, *Austrian Economics and the Political Economy of Freedom* (Northhampton, MA: Edward Elgar, 2003).

23. Frank H. Knight, "Economic History," in Philip P. Wiener, editor, *Dictionary of the History of Ideas*, 4 vols. (New York: Scribner's, 1973), vol. 2, pp. 44-61; p. 50, emphasis in the original.

24. http://www.nobel.se/economics/laureates/1970/

25. Nobel Prize in Economic Sciences Winners 2002-1969. http://almaz.com/nobel/economics/economics.html

26. See chapter 4.

27. Quoted in Alan Ebenstein, *Friedrich Hayek: A Biography* (New York: Palgrave, 2001), p. 261.

28. "Modern Portfolio Theory," http://www.moneychimp.com/articles/risk/riskintro.htm.

29. See Hans-Hermann Hoppe, *A Theory of Socialism and Capitalism: Economics, Politics, and Ethics* (Boston: Kluwer Academic Publishers, 1989), chapter 7.

30. Sylvia Nasar, *A Beautiful Mind: The Life of Mathematical Genius and Nobel Laureate John Nash* (New York: Simon and Schuster, 1998).

31. John F. Nash, Jr., "Autobiography," *Les Prix Nobel 1994*; http://www.nobel.se/economics/laureates/1994/nash-autobio.html, emphasis added.

32. http://www.nobel.se/economics/laureates/2002/press.html

33. Daniel Altman, "A Nobel that bridges economics and psychology," *New York Times*, October 10, 2002, p. C1, emphasis added.

34. Joshua Tauberer, "Kahneman wins Nobel Prize in economics for behavioral study," *Daily Princetonian*, October 10, 2002. http://www.dailyprincetonian.com/archives/2002/10/10/news/5684.shtml, emphasis added.

35. Justin Fox, "Is the market rational: No, say the experts. But neither are you, so don't go thinking you can outsmart it," *Fortune*, December 9, 2002, pp. 117-126; p. 118.

36. Ibid., p. 120.

37. Ibid., p. 124.

38. Ibid., emphasis added.

39. Sigmund Freud, *The Psychopathology of Everyday Life* [1901], in *The Standard Edition of the Complete Psychological Works of Sigmund Freud*, translated by James Strachey, 24 vols. (London: Hogarth Press, 1953-1974), volume 6.

40. From Nobel Lectures, Physiology or Medicine 1942-1962. http://www.nobel.se/medicine/laureates/1949/press.html, emphasis added.

41. "Lobotomy's hall of fame," http://www.epub.org.br/cm/n02/historia/important.htm.

42. Thomas Szasz, *Schizophrenia: The Sacred Symbol of Psychiatry* [1976] (Syracuse: Syracuse University Press, 1988), chapter 3.

43. The Noble Assembly, Karolinska Institute, "Press release," October 9, 2000. http://www.nobel.se/medicine/laureates/2000/press.html

44. Ibid., emphasis added.

45. Eric R. Kandel, "Autobiography," http://www.nobel.se/medicine/laureates/2000/kandel-autobio.html.

46. The Noble Assembly, Karolinska Institute, "Press release," October 9, 2000. http://www.nobel.se/medicine/laureates/2000/press.html

47. Eric R. Kandel, "A new intellectual framework for psychiatry," *American Journal of Psychiatry*, 155: 457-469 (April), 1998. http://www.hhmi.org/bulletin/kandel/, emphasis added.

48. Theodor Meynert, *Psychiatry: Clinical Treatise on Diseases of the Forebrain* [1884], translated by B. Sachs (New York: G. P. Putnam's Sons, 1885), p. v, emphasis in the original.
49. Steve Mirsky, "The future of psychiatry: Eric Kandel says it lies with biology," reprinted from the September 2000 *HHMI Bulletin*, Vol. 13, No. 3, pp. 6-8. http://www.hhmi.org/bulletin/kandel/
50. Eric R. Kandel, "A new intellectual framework for psychiatry," *American Journal of Psychiatry*, 155: 457-469 (April), 1998. http://www.hhmi.org/bulletin/kandel/, emphasis added.
51. Jamie Talan, "Thinking beyond the Nobel: 3 scientists turn talents to setting up biotech companies," *Newsday*, June 16, 2003. http://www.newsday.com/business/local/newyork/ny-bzcov163334257jun16,0,626692.story
52. Quoted in James C. Marshall, "The nerve cells of the soul," *New York Times Book Review*, January 16, 1994, p. 24.
53. "Neuroeconomics," June 7, 2003, http://www.quinion.com/words/turnsofphrase/tp-neu3.htm.
54. Sandra Blakeslee, "Brain experts now follow the money," *New York Times*, June 17, 2003. http://college4.nytimes.com/guests/articles/2003/06/17/2108703.xml, emphasis added.
55. Sharon Begley, "Scientists study how we think about money," *Wall Street Journal Europe*, November 15, 2002, p. A6, emphasis added.
56. Virginia Postrel, "Looking inside the brains of the stingy," *New York Times,* February 27, 2003. http://www.nytimes.com/2003/02/27/business/27SCEN.html, emphasis added.
57. Lise Menn, "Neurolinguistics," http://www.lsadc.org/Menn.html.
58. Thomas Szasz, *Ceremonial Chemistry*, op. cit.
59. Thomas Szasz, *Pharmacracy: Medicine and Politics in America* [2001] (Syracuse: Syracuse University Press, 2003).

Chapter 4. Economocracy and Pharmacracy

1. Adam Smith, *Lectures on Justice, Police, Revenue, and Arms* [1763/1896], quoted in Edwin G. West, *Adam Smith* (Indianapolis: Liberty Press, 1976), p. 87.
2. Adam Smith, *The Theory of Moral Sentiments* [1759] (Indianapolis, IN: Liberty Classics, 1976), p. 78; see also Bernard Bailyn, *To Begin the World Anew: The Genius and Ambiguities of the American Founders* (New York: Knopf, 2003).
3. Edmund Burke, "A letter from Mr. Burke to a Member of the National Assembly in answer to some objections to his book on French Affairs" [1791], in *The Works of the Right Honorable Edmund Burke*, 12 vols. (Boston: Wells & Lilly, 1826), vol. 3, p. 315.
4. Adam Smith, *Lectures on Justice*, op. cit., p. 79.
5. Jennifer Roback Morse, *Love & Economics: Why the Laissez-Faire Family Doesn't Work* (Dallas, Pence Publishing Company, 2001), p. 28.
6. Thomas Szasz, *Cruel Compassion: The Psychiatric Control of Society's Unwanted* [1994] (Syracuse: Syracuse University Press, 1998).
7. Kenneth Minogue, "Pisher's progress," *National Review*, December 31, 1989, pp. 38-39; p. 38.
8. See Thomas Szasz, *Ceremonial Chemistry: The Ritual Persecution of Drugs, Addicts, and Pushers* [1976] (Syracuse: Syracuse University Press, 2003); *Cruel Compassion*, op. cit.; *Our Right to Drugs: The Case for a Free Market* [1992] (Syracuse: Syracuse University Press, 1996); *Pharmacracy: Medicine and Politics*

in America [2001] (Syracuse: Syracuse University Press, 2003); and *Liberation By Oppression: A Comparative Study of Slavery and Psychiatry* (New Brunswick, NJ: Transaction Publishers, 2002).

9.   Ludwig von Mises, *Human Action: A Treatise on Economics* (New Haven: Yale University Press, 1949), p. 729.

10.   Thomas Szasz, "The myth of mental illness," *American Psychologist*, 15: 113-118 (February), 1960; and *The Myth of Mental Illness: Foundations of a Theory of Personal Conduct* [1961], revised edition (New York: HarperCollins, 1974).

11.   Thomas Szasz, *Law, Liberty, and Psychiatry: An Inquiry Into the Social Uses of Mental Health Practices* [1963] (Syracuse: Syracuse University Press, 1989), pp. 212-222.

12.   Thomas Szasz, *Ceremonial Chemistry*, op. cit., p. 139.

13.   Wilhelm Röpke, *A Humane Economy: The Special Framework of the Free Market* (Indianapolis: Liberty Fund, 1971), p. 283.

14.   Thomas Szasz, *Ceremonial Chemistry*, op. cit.; *Pharmacracy*, op. cit.; *Liberation By Oppression*, op. cit. See also, Charlotte Twight, *Dependent on D.C.: The Rise of Federal Control Over the Lives of Ordinary Americans* (New York: St. Martin's Press/Palgrave, 2002).

15.   Quoted in, *The Great Quotations*, compiled by George Seldes (New York: Lyle Stuart, 1960), p. 354.

16.   Helmut Schoeck, *Envy: A Theory of Social Behaviour* [1966], translated by Michael Glenny and Betty Ross (New York: Harcourt, Brace & World, 1969).

17.   Peter T. Bauer, *Reality and Rhetoric: Studies in Economic Development* (London: Weidenfeld and Nicolson, 1984), p. 158. See also Paul E. Gottfried, *Multiculturalism and the Politics of Guilt* (Columbia, MO: University of Missouri Press, 2002); *After Liberalism: Mass Democracy in the Managerial State* (Princeton: Princeton University Press, 2001).

18.   http://www.sharedcapitalism.org/, emphasis added.

19.   Jeff Gates, "Is persistent abject poverty now a policy choice?" *Society*, 4; 20-27 (July/August), 2003, p. 20, emphasis added.

20.   Ibid., p. 22, emphasis added.

21.   Ibid., p. 27, emphasis added.

22.   John McKenzie, "The global airliner," *Baltimore Sun*, April 14, 2002. http://www. backpacknation.org/sun_article.shtml

23.   Thomas Szasz, *Words to the Wise: A Medical-Philosophical Dictionary* (New Brunswick, NJ: Transaction Publishers, 2004), pp. 65-78.

24.   Thomas Szasz, *Liberation By Oppression*, op. cit. and *Words to the Wise*, op. cit.

25.   Peter Bauer, "Foreign aid" [1996], in *From Subsistence to Exchange and other Essays* (Princeton: Princeton University Press, 2000), pp. 41-52; p. 42.

26.   Peter T. Bauer, *Dissent on Development: Studies and Debates in Development*, revised edition (Cambridge: Harvard University Press, 1976), p. 115.

27.   Ibid., p. 112.

28.   Thomas Szasz, *Ceremonial Chemistry*, op. cit.

29.   Peter T. Bauer, *Dissent on Development*, op. cit., p. 96.

30.   http://www.imf.org/external/about.htm

31.   World Bank. http://web.worldbank.org/WBSITE/EXTERNAL/EXTABOUTUS/ 0,pagePK:43912~piPK:36602,00.html

32.   Thomas Szasz, *Cruel Compassion*, op. cit.

33.   Peter Bauer, quoted in "A voice for the poor," *The Economist* (Print Edition), May 2, 2002.

34.   See James A. Dorn, Steven H. Hanke, and Alan A. Walters, editors, *The Revolution in Development Economics* (Washington, D. C.: Cato Institute, 1998).

35.   James M. Buchanan, *What Should Economists Do?* (Indianapolis: Liberty Press, 1979), pp. 26-27, emphasis in the original. The term "catallactics" was first proposed by the English economist Richard Whateley (1787-1863), and was used by Ludwig von Mises, *Human Action*, op. cit., p. 3. Symbiosis, borrowed from biology, is a familiar term.

36.   Ibid., p. 31, emphasis added.

37.   Ibid., p. 34, emphasis added.

38.   See chapter 2.

39.   James M. Buchanan, *What Should Economists Do?* op. cit., p. 39, emphasis in the original.

40.   Ibid., p. 47.

41.   Ibid., p. 84.

42.   Ibid., p. 85.

43.   Ibid., pp. 64, 279. The allusion is to Hayek's essay, "Why I Am Not a Conservative," in Friedrich A. Hayek, *The Constitution of Liberty* (Chicago: University of Chicago Press, 1960), pp. 397-411.

44.   Edmund Burke, *Reflections on the Revolution in France* [1790], Foreword by Francis Canavan (Indianapolis: Liberty Fund, 1999), pp. 127-128.

45.   Kofi Annan, quoted in "Editorial," *National Catholic Reporter*, March 29, 2002. http://www.natcath.com/NCR_Online/archives/032902/032902n.htm

46.   Edmund Burke, *Reflections on the Revolution in France*, op. cit., p. 362.

47.   Quoted in *The Oxford Dictionary of Political Quotations*, edited by Anthony Jay (New York: Oxford University Press, 1996), p. 68.

48.   Mortimer J. Adler, *The Idea of Freedom*, 2 vols. (Garden City, NY: Doubleday, 1958-1961).

49.   Thomas Szasz, *Liberation By Oppression*, op. cit.

50.   John Locke, *Two Treatises on Government* [1690], edited by Peter Laslett (New York: New American Library, 1965).

51.   "The Philosopher of Freedom," http://www.blupete.com/Literature/Biographies/Philosophy/Locke.htm.

52.   James Madison, "Federalist, No. 10," http://www.systemsoap.com/get/itnowbas2.php?yhgeouspu2_itnowbas.

53.   *Popular Government*, at Sir Henry Sumner Maine, http://www.blupete.com/Literature/Biographies/Law/Maine.htm. For modern support of this contention, see Hans-Hermann Hoppe, *"Democracy—The God That Failed: The Economics and Politics of Monarchy, Democracy, and Natural Order"* (New Brunswick, NJ: Transaction Publishers, 2001).

54.   Henry Sumner Maine, *Ancient Law: Its Connection With the Early History of Society, and Its Relation to Modern Ideas* [1864], Foreword by Lawrence Rosen (Tucson: University of Arizona Press, 1986), pp. 163-165, emphasis added.

Chapter 5. John Stuart Mill

1.   Karl Britton, *John Stuart Mill* (London: Penguin, 1953), p. 10.

2.   John Stuart Mill, *Autobiography* [1873], in *Essential Works of John Stuart Mill*, edited by Max Lerner (New York: Bantam Books, 1961), pp. 1-182; p. 55.

3.   Daniel Defoe, "Demand for public control of madhouses" [1728], in Thomas Szasz, editor, *The Age of Madness: A History of Involuntary Mental Hospitalization Presented in Selected Texts* (Garden City, NY: Anchor Press/Doubleday, 1973), pp. 7-8.

4.   John Stuart Mill, "The Law of Lunacy," *Daily News*, July 31, 1858, p. 4, in, *Collected Works of John Stuart Mill*, edited by Ann P. Robson and John M. Brown, 25 vols. (Toronto: University of Toronto Press, 1986), vol. 24, p. 1198-1199.

5.   John Stuart Mill, *On Liberty* [1859] (Chicago: Regnery, 1955), p. 14.

6.   Ibid., p. 18, emphasis added.

7.   Ibid., p. 14.

8.   Quoted in Henry A. Foley and Steven S. Sharfstein, *Madness and Government: Who Cares for the Mentally Ill?* (Washington, DC: American Psychiatric Press, 1983), p. vii. In this connection, see Thomas Szasz, *Pharmacracy: Medicine and Politics in America* [2001] (Syracuse: Syracuse University Press, 2003).

9.   John Stuart Mill, *On Liberty*, op. cit., pp. 99-100, emphasis added.

10.   Ibid., pp. 111-112, 115.

11.   Ibid., pp. 118-119, 120.

12.   Ibid., pp. 120-121, 124.

13.   Ibid., pp. 141-143, 145-146, emphasis added.

14.   Ibid., 161.

15.   Thomas Szasz, *Insanity: The Idea and Its Consequences* [1987] (Syracuse: Syracuse University Press, 1997).

16.   James Fitzjames Stephen, *Liberty, Equality, Fraternity* [1874], *and Three Brief Essays*, Foreword by Richard A. Posner (Chicago: University of Chicago Press, 1991), pp. 68-69. For further discussion, see Thomas Szasz, *Insanity*, op. cit. and *Cruel Compassion: The Psychiatric Control of Society's Unwanted* [1994] (Syracuse University Press, 1998).

17.   Milton Friedman, *Capitalism and Freedom* (Chicago: University of Chicago Press, 1962), p. 33.

18.   See Thomas Szasz, *The Myth of Mental Illness: Foundations of a Theory of Personal Conduct* [1961], revised edition (New York: Harper & Row, 1974); *Law, Liberty, and Psychiatry* [1963] (Syracuse: Syracuse University Press, 1989); *Psychiatric Justice* [1965] (Syracuse: Syracuse University Press, 1988); *The Age of Madness*, op. cit.; *Insanity*, op. cit.

19.   John Stuart Mill, *Utilitarianism* [1863], in *Essential Works of John Stuart Mill*, edited by Max Lerner (New York: Bantam Books, 1961), pp. 189-252; p. 194.

20.   Ibid., p. 208.

21.   Ibid., p. 204.

22.   Linda Raeder, *John Stuart Mill and the Religion of Humanity* (Columbia, MO: University of Missouri Press, 2002), pp. 320-322, 342.

23.   John Stuart Mill, *The Subjection of Women* [1869], Introduction by Wendell Robert Carr (Cambridge: MIT Press, 1970).

24.   John Stuart Mill, *Utilitarianism*, op. cit., p. 247.

25.   Ibid., pp. 247-248.

Chapter 6. Bertrand Russell

1.   *Encyclopaedia Britannica*, 16th edition, 1966, vol. 9, p. 769.

2.   Bertrand Russell, *The Conquest of Happiness* (New York: Horace Liveright, 1930), p. 17.

3.   Ibid., p. 198.

4.   Bertrand Russell, *Roads to Freedom: Socialism, Anarchism, and Syndicalism* [1918] (London: George Allen and Unwin, 1966).

5.   Ibid., pp. 126, 133.

6.   Ibid., p. 127.

7.   Bertrand Russell, "John Stuart Mill" [1951], in *Portraits from Memory*, reprinted in Jerome B. Schneewind, editor, *Mill: A Collection of Critical Essays* (Garden City, NY: Anchor Books, 1968), pp. 1-21; p. 20.
8.   Bertrand Russell, *Roads to Freedom*, op. cit., pp. 129-130.
9.   Ibid., p. 134.
10.   Ibid., p. 91.
11.   Ibid., pp. 127-128.
12.   Ibid., pp. 86, 135; and see Franz Alexander and Hugo Staub, *The Criminal, the Judge, and the Public: A Psychological Analysis* [1929], translated by Gregory Zilboorg (Glencoe, Ill: The Free Press and the Falcon's Wing Press, 1956) and Karl Menninger, *The Crime of Punishment* (New York: Viking, 1968).
13.   Bertrand Russell, *Roads to Freedom*, op. cit., pp. 89, 90, 86-87, 130, emphasis added.
14.   Thomas Szasz, *Law, Liberty, and Psychiatry: An Inquiry Into the Social Uses of Mental Health Practices* [1963] (Syracuse: Syracuse University Press, 1989); *The Manufacture of Madness: A Comparative Study of the Inquisition and the Mental Health Movement* [1970] (Syracuse: Syracuse University Press, 1997); *The Therapeutic State: Psychiatry in the Mirror of Current Events* (Buffalo: Prometheus Books, 1984); *Insanity: The Idea and Its Consequences* [1987] (Syracuse: Syracuse University Press, 1997); *Cruel Compassion: The Psychiatric Control of Society's Unwanted* [1994] (Syracuse: Syracuse University Press, 1998); and *Pharmacracy: Medicine and Politics in America* [2001] (Syracuse: Syracuse University Press, 2003).
15.   Quoted in Ray Monk, *Bertrand Russell: The Ghosts of Madness, 1921-1970* (New York: Free Press, 2001), p. 15.
16.   Ibid., pp. 104-105.
17.   Ibid., p. 105, emphasis added.
18.   Ibid., p. 106.
19.   Bertrand Russell, *The Conquest of Happiness*, op. cit., p. 111.
20.   Bertrand Russell, *Power: A New Social Analysis* (London: George Allen & Unwin, 1938), p. 270.
21.   Thomas Szasz, *Schizophrenia: The Sacred Symbol of Psychiatry* [1976] (Syracuse: Syracuse University Press, 1988).
22.   Thomas Szasz, *Insanity*, op. cit.
23.   Bertrand Russell, *Power*, op. cit., p. 9.
24.   Quoted in Ray Monk, *Bertrand Russell*, op. cit., pp. 9-10.
25.   Ibid., pp. 99-100.
26.   Ibid., p. 100.
27.   Ibid., p. 95.
28.   Ibid., p. 359.
29.   Ibid., p. 362.
30.   Ibid.
31.   Thomas Szasz, "The psychiatric will: A new mechanism for protecting persons against 'psychosis' and psychiatry," *American Psychologist*, 37: 762-770 (July), 1982; and *Liberation By Oppression: A Comparative Study of Slavery and Psychiatry* (New Brunswick, NJ: Transaction Publishers, 2002), chapters 5 and 6.
32.   Ray Monk, *Bertrand Russell*, op. cit., p. 363.
33.   Ibid., pp. 363-364, emphasis added.
34.   Ibid., p. 366.
35.   Ibid., p. 491.
36.   Ibid., p. 500.
37.   Ibid., p. 484.

38. See Thomas Szasz, *The Myth of Mental Illness: Foundations of a theory of personal conduct* [1961], revised edition (New York: HarperCollins, 1974); *The Manufacture of Madness*, op. cit.; *Insanity*, op. city.; *Cruel Compassion*, op. cit.; and Thomas Szasz, editor, *The Age of Madness: A History of Involuntary Mental Hospitalization Presented in Selected Texts* (Garden City, NY: Doubleday Anchor, 1973).

39. Herbert G. Wells, *The Island of Doctor Moreau: A Possibility*, 1896. http://www.literature.org/authors/wells-herbert-george/the-island-of-doctor-moreau/chapter-22.html

40. See Thomas Szasz, "*Ex Parte* Psychiatry," in Thomas Szasz, *A Lexicon of Lunacy: Metaphoric Malady, Personal Responsibility, and Psychiatry* (New Brunswick: Transaction Publishers, 1993), pp. 173-185.

41. Thomas Szasz, *The Manufacture of Madness*, op. cit., chapter 11.

42. Ray Monk, *Bertrand Russell*, op. cit., p. 359.

43. Ibid., p. 370.

44. See Daniel Defoe, "Demand for public control of madhouses" [1728], in Thomas Szasz, editor, *The Age of Madness*, op. cit., pp. 7-9.

45. For another example of the literary recognition of the parts played by both patient and doctor in the evils of mad-doctoring, see Virginia Woolf, *Mrs. Dalloway* [1925] (New York: Harcourt, Brace & World, 1953).

46. Bertrand Russell, *Satan in the Suburbs, and Other Stories* (New York: Simon and Schuster, 1953). He also wrote another collection of short stories: *Nightmares of Eminent Persons, and Other Stories* [1954] (Harmondsworth: Penguin, 1962).

47. Bertrand Russell, *Satan in the Suburbs*, op. cit., p. vii.

48. Ibid., pp. 1-59; p. 37.

49. Ibid., p. 56.

50. Ibid., 56-57.

51. Ibid., p. 59.

52. Bertrand Russell, "The psycho-analyst's nightmare: Adjustment—a fugue," in Bertrand Russell, *Nightmares of Eminent Persons, and Other Stories*, op. cit., pp. 27-37; p. 36.

53. Bertrand Russell, "Introduction: On the Value of Scepticism," in Bertrand Russell, *Sceptical Essays* (London: Allen & Unwin, 1928), http://www.mcmaster.ca/russdocs/brquotes.htm.

54. Bertrand Russell, "The infra-redioscope," in Bertrand Russell, *Satan in the Suburbs*, op. cit., pp. 87-117.

55. Ibid., p. 112, emphasis added.

56. Ibid., pp. 116-117.

57. Bertrand Russell, "The Guardians of Parnassus," in ibid., pp. 118-131; pp. 130-131.

Chapter 7. The American Civil Liberties Union

1. http://216.239.39.100 search?q=cache:cJZ5UQHD2wYC:www.aclu.org/library/FreedomIsWhy.pdf+aclu+history&hl=en&ie=UTF-8

2. Charles L. Markmann, *The Noblest Cry: A History of the American Civil Liberties Union* (New York: St. Martin's Press, 1965), p. 400.

3. See Thomas Szasz, "The ACLU's mental illness cop-out," *Reason*, January 1974, pp. 4-9; reprinted in Thomas Szasz, *The Therapeutic State: Psychiatry in the Mirror of Current Events* (Buffalo: Prometheus Books, 1984), pp. 58-66.

4. Charles L. Markmann, cited in Thomas Szasz, "The ACLU's mental illness cop-out," in Thomas Szasz, *The Therapeutic State*, op. cit., p. 63.

5. See especially Thomas Szasz, *Law, Liberty, and Psychiatry: An Inquiry into the Social Uses of Psychiatry* [1963] (Syracuse: Syracuse University Press, 1989); *The Manufacture of Madness: A Comparative Study of the Inquisition and the Mental Health Movement* [1970] (Syracuse: Syracuse University Press, 1997); *Ceremonial Chemistry: The Ritual Persecution of Drugs, Addicts, and Pushers* [1976] (Syracuse: Syracuse University Press, 2003); *Cruel Compassion: The Psychiatric Control of Society's Unwanted* [1994] (Syracuse: Syracuse University Press, 1998); *The Therapeutic State*, op. cit.; *Our Right to Drugs: The Case for a Free Market* [1992] (Syracuse: Syracuse University Press, 1996); *Pharmacracy: Medicine and Politics in America* [2001] (Syracuse: Syracuse University Press, 2003); and *Liberation By Oppression: A Comparative Study of Slavery and Psychiatry* (New Brunswick, NJ: Transaction Publishers, 2002).

6. Charles L. Markmann, cited in Thomas Szasz, *The Therapeutic State*, op. cit., p. 65.

7. Thomas Szasz, *Cruel Compassion*, op. cit.

8. Thomas Szasz, *Liberation By Oppression*, op. cit.

9. Aryeh Neier, cited in Thomas Szasz, "Condoning psychiatric slavery," *Inquiry*, March 6, 1978, pp. 3-4; reprinted in Thomas Szasz, *The Therapeutic State*, op. cit., pp. 69-73; p. 70.

10. Karl Menninger, cited in Thomas Szasz, *The Therapeutic State*, op. cit., pp. 59-60.

11. "International Action Center," http://www.iacenter.org/. See also, Anthony York, "Ramsey Clark, the war criminal's best friend," *Salon.com*, June 18, 1999. http://www.salon.com/news/feature/1999/06/21/clark/

12. Ramsey Clark, cited in Thomas Szasz, *The Therapeutic State*, op. cit., p. 60, emphasis added.

13. See Thomas Szasz, *Fatal Freedom: The Ethics and Politics of Suicide* [1999] (Syracuse: Syracuse University Press, 2002) and *Pharmacracy*, op. cit.

14. Aryeh Neier, *Taking Liberties: Four Decades in the Struggle for Rights* (New York: Public Affairs, 2003), p. 50, emphasis added.

15. Thomas Szasz, *Insanity: The Idea and Its Consequences* [1987] (Syracuse: Syracuse University Press, 1997).

16. Gerald Grob, "American Psychiatry," in Hugh Freeman, editor, *A Century of Psychiatry* (London: Mosby-Wolfe/Harcourt Publishers, 1999), pp. 195-201; p. 201.

17. Kathleen Jones, "The Diminishing Mental Hospitals," in Ibid., pp. 191-195; p. 193, emphasis added.

18. Ronald D. Laing, *The Divided Self: An Existential Study in Sanity and Madness* (London: Tavistock Publications, 1960), p. 27, emphasis added.

19. Ronald D. Laing, "Round the bend" (Review of Szasz, T. S., *The Theology of Medicine*, *The Myth of Psychotherapy*, and *Schizophrenia*), *New Statesman*, July 20, 1979, pp. 96-97, emphasis in the original.

20. Anthony Stadlen, "Dropping the medical metaphor" (Letters), *New Statesman*, August 17, 1979, pp. 236-237.

21. John Clay, *R. D. Laing: A Divided Self* (London: Hodder & Stoughton, 1996), p. 181.

22. Thomas Szasz, "Mental illness: Psychiatry's phlogiston," *Journal of Medical Ethics*, 27: 297-301 (October), 2001.

23. Charles L. Markmann, cited in Thomas Szasz, "Condoning psychiatric slavery," in *The Therapeutic State*, op. cit., p. 72.

24. Robert M. Levy and Leonard S. Rubenstein, *The Rights of People with Mental Disabilities: The Authoritative ACLU Guide to the Rights of People with Mental Illness and Mental Retardation* (Carbondale, IL: Southern Illinois University Press, 1996).
25. Ibid., p. 1.
26. Frederick Douglass, "What the Black Man Wants," in Howard Brotz, editor, *Negro Social and Political Thought 1850-1920: Representative Texts* (New York: Basic Books, Inc. 1962), p. 283, emphasis added.
27. Robert M. Levy and Leonard S. Rubenstein, *The Rights of People with Mental Disabilities*, op. cit., p. 13, emphasis added.
28. Thomas Szasz, *Psychiatric Slavery: When Confinement and Coercion Masquerade as Cure* [1977] (Syracuse: Syracuse University Press, 1998), *Liberation By Oppression*, op. cit., and Thomas Szasz, editor, *The Age of Madness: A History of Involuntary Mental Hospitalization Presented in Selected Texts* (Garden City, NY: Doubleday Anchor, 1973).
29. Robert M. Levy and Leonard S. Rubenstein, *The Rights of People with Mental Disabilities*, op. cit., pp. 15, 205, emphasis added.
30. Ibid., 215, emphasis added.
31. Ibid., p. 215.
32. Ibid., p. 309.
33. See for example, Susan Welsh and Martin P. Deahl, "Modern psychiatric ethics," *The Lancet*, 359: 253-55 (19 January) 2002. http://www.thelancet.com/journal/vol/iss/full/llan.359.9302.editorial_and_re; Bradford E Young, "Evidence: 'Dangerous patient' exception to psychotherapist-patient privilege," *American Journal of Law and Medicine*, 28: 514-516 (2002). Even Freud reserved the privilege of betraying his patient's confidences: "I make use of his [patient's] communication without asking his consent, since I cannot allow that psychoanalytic technique has any right to claim the protection of medical discretion." Sigmund Freud, "On the history of the psychoanalytic movement" [1914], *The Standard Edition of the Complete Psychological Works of Sigmund Freud*, translated by James Strachey, 24 vols. (London: Hogarth Press, 1953-1974), vol. 14, pp. 1-66; p. 64.
34. Robert M. Levy and Leonard S. Rubenstein, *The Rights of People with Mental Disabilities*, op. cit., p. 299, emphasis added.
35. Ibid., p. 49, emphasis added.
36. Ibid., pp. 302-303, emphasis added.
37. In this connection, see Thomas Szasz, "American Association for the Abolition of Involuntary Mental Hospitalization," *American Journal of Psychiatry*, 127: 1698 (June), 1971; "The American Association for the Abolition of Involuntary Mental Hospitalization," *Abolitionist*, 1: 1-2 (Summer), 1971; "A.A.A.I.M.H.—R.I.P.," *Abolitionist*, 9: 1 & 4 (September), 1979.
38. Robert M. Levy and Leonard S. Rubenstein, *The Rights of People with Mental Disabilities*, op. cit., pp. 21-24.
39. http://archive.aclu.org/library/ibrights.html
40. Quoted in Thomas Szasz, *Law, Liberty, and Psychiatry*, op. cit., p. 61.

Chapter 8. Ayn Rand

1. http://www.aynrand.org/. For an outstanding biography of Rand, see Chris Matthew Sciabarra, *Ayn Rand: The Russian Radical* (University Park, PA: Pennsylvania State University Press, 1995).

2.   Murray Rothbard, "The Sociology of the Ayn Rand Cult" (1972), http://www. lewrockwell.com/rothbard/rothbard23.html. Copyright © 2003 by the Ludwig von Mises Institute. Further quotes are from this source.

3.   Thomas Szasz, *The Myth of Psychotherapy: Mental Healing as Religion, Rhetoric, and Repression* [1978] (Syracuse: Syracuse University Press, 1988).

4.   Thomas Szasz, *Heresies* (Garden City, NY: Anchor Doubleday, 1976), p. 137.

5.   Thomas Szasz, *Words to the Wise: A Medical-Philosophical Dictionary* (New Brunswick, NJ: Transaction Publishers, 2004), p. 174.

6.   Thomas Szasz, *The Second Sin* (New York: Anchor Doubleday, 1974), p. 79.

7.   Ayn Rand, *Letters of Ayn Rand,* edited by Michael S. Berliner, introduction by Leonard Peikoff (New York: E. P. Dutton, 1995), p. 506.

8.   Ibid., p. 513, emphasis in the original.

9.   Ibid., p. 514.

10.   Ibid.

11.   Ibid., pp. 522.

12.   Ibid., p. 524.

13.   Ibid., pp. 545-546.

14.   Ibid., p. 559, emphasis added.

15.   Ibid., pp. 559-560.

16.   Ibid., p. 560, emphasis added.

17.   Justin Raimondo, *An Enemy of the State: The Life of Murray N. Rothbard* (Amherst, NY: Prometheus Books, 2000), p. 110.

18.   Ibid., p. 115.

19.   Whittaker Chambers, "Big sister is watching you," *National Review*, December 28, 1957, pp. 594-596. http://www.potomac-inc.org/aynrand.html

20.   Chris Matthew Sciabarra, *Ayn Rand*, op. cit.

21.   Chris Matthew Sciabarra, personal communication, email dated March 25, 2003.

22.   Ayn Rand, *Letters*, op. cit., p. 559, emphasis added.

23.   Chris Matthew Sciabarra, *Ayn Rand*, op. cit., p. 200.

24.   American Psychiatric Association, *Diagnostic and Statistical Manual of Mental Disorders—IV*, 4th edition (Washington, D.C.: American Psychiatric Association, 1994).

25.   Ralph Waldo Emerson, *Journal L.,* http://www.geocities.com/Athens/Parthe-non/5658/introen.html; also http://www.mimno.net/html/intuition.html.

Chapter 9. Nathaniel Branden

1.   http://www.nathanielbranden.net

2.   Charles S. Peirce, "How to Make Our Ideas Clear" [1878], in *Values in a Universe of Chance: Selected Writings of Charles S. Peirce (1839-1914)*, edited by Philip P. Wiener (Garden City, NY: Doubleday Anchor, 1958), pp. 113-136; p. 124.

3.   Nathaniel Branden, *The Psychology of Self-Esteem: A New Concept of Man's Psychological Nature* (Los Angeles: Nash, 1969).

4.   Ibid., p. ix.

5.   Ibid., emphasis added.

6.   Ibid., p. 35, emphasis added.

7.   Ibid., p. 26, emphasis in the original.

8.   Ibid., p. 89, emphasis added.

9.   Ibid., pp. 91-92.

10.   Ibid., p. 92.

11.   Ibid., p. 93, emphasis in the original.

12. Ibid., p. 94, emphasis in the original.
13. Ibid., p. 95, emphasis added.
14. Ibid., p. 167, emphasis in the original.
15. Ibid., p. 193.
16. Ibid., p. 196.
17. Ibid., p. 103.
18. Ibid., pp. 213-214, 225, emphasis added.
19. Ibid., p. 228.
20. Ibid., p. 230.
21. See generally Thomas Szasz, *The Myth of Psychotherapy: Mental Healing as Religion, Rhetoric, and Repression* [1978] (Syracuse: Syracuse University Press, 1988).
22. Jim Powell, *The Triumph of Liberty: A 2,000-Year History, Told Through the Lives of Freedom's Greatest Champions* (New York: Free Press, 2000), p. 345.
23. Nathaniel Branden, *Breaking Free* (Los Angeles: Nash, 1970), pp. 10-11.
24. Ibid., p. vi.
25. Ibid., p. 9.
26. Ibid., p. 209.
27. Ibid., p. 210.
28. See Thomas Szasz, *Insanity: The Idea and Its Consequences* [1987] (Syracuse: Syracuse University Press, 1997) and *Cruel Compassion: The Psychiatric Control of Society's Unwanted* [1994] (Syracuse: Syracuse University Press, 1998).
29. Nathaniel Branden, "Break free! An interview with Nathaniel Branden," *Reason*, October 1971, pp. 4-19; pp. 6-7.
30. Ibid., p. 7.
31. Thomas Szasz, *The Ethics of Psychoanalysis: The Theory and Method of Autonomous Psychotherapy* [1965] (Syracuse: Syracuse University Press, 1988); *The Myth of Psychotherapy*, op. cit.; "The cure of souls in the therapeutic state," *The Psychoanalytic Review*, 90: 45-62 (February) 2003; "Cleansing the modern heart," *Society*, 40: 52-59 (May/June), 2003.
32. Richard Weaver, *Ideas Have Consequences* (Chicago: University of Chicago Press/Phoenix Books, 1962).
33. Thomas Szasz, *Insanity*, op. cit.
34. Thomas Szasz, *Pharmacracy: Medicine and Politics in America* [2001] (Syracuse: Syracuse University Press, 2003), chapter 4.
35. Nathaniel Branden, *Judgment Day: My Years With Ayn Rand* (Boston: Houghton Mifflin, 1989), p. 16.
36. Ibid., p. 220, emphasis added.
37. Ibid., p. 156.
38. Ibid., p. 137, emphasis in the original.
39. Ibid., p. 126.
40. Ibid., p. 166.
41. Ibid., p. 167, emphasis added.
42. Barbara Branden, *The Passion of Ayn Rand* (New York: Doubleday, 1986), pp. 276-277.
43. Ibid., p. 277, emphasis added.
44. Nathaniel Branden, *Judgment Day*, op. cit., pp. 167, 169, emphasis added.
45. Ibid., p. 256.
46. Ibid., p. 346, emphasis added.
47. Ibid., p. 296
48. Ibid., p. 347.
49. Ibid., pp. 347-348, emphasis added.

50. Ibid., p. 372, emphasis added.
51. Ibid., p. 423.
52. Ibid., pp. 423-424.
53. "Full Context Interview with Nathaniel Branden," by Karen Reedstrom. Copyright © 1996, Full Context, reproduced by permission.http://www.vix.com/objectiv-ism/Writing/NathanielBranden/FullContextInterview.html
54. Ibid.
55. Justin Raimondo, *An Enemy of the State: The Life of Murray N. Rothbard* (Amherst, NY: Prometheus Books, 2000).
56. Ibid., pp. 123, 122.
57. Ibid., p. 124.
58. Ibid., p. 130.
59. Ibid., emphasis added.
60. Email from Justin Raimondo to Thomas Szasz, May 5, 2003.
61. Justin Raimondo, *An Enemy of the State*, op. cit., p. 128.
62. Ibid, pp. 128, 129.
63. Nathaniel Branden, *Judgment Day*, op. cit., p. 95.
64. Quoted in Jeff Walker, *The Ayn Rand Cult* (Chicago: Open Court, 1999), pp. 151, 169.

Chapter 10. Ludwig von Mises

1. Cited in Alan Ebenstein, *Friedrich Hayek: A Biography* (New York: Palgrave, 2001), p. 36.
2. Ludwig von Mises, *The Theory of Money and Credit* [1912], translated by H. E. Bateson (Indianapolis: LibertyClassics, 1980).
3. Ludwig von Mises, *Socialism: An Economic and Sociological Analysis* [1922], translated by J. Kahane (Indianapolis: Liberty Fund, 1981).
4. http://www.mises.org/mises.asp
5. http://www.mises.org/
6. http://www.mises.org/mises.asp
7. Ludwig von Mises, *Human Action: A Treatise on Economics* (New Haven: Yale University Press, 1949), p. 3.
8. Ludwig von Mises, *Socialism*, op. cit, p. 107.
9. Ludwig von Mises, *Human Action: A Treatise on Economics*, fourth revised edition (Irvington-on-Hudson, NY: Foundation for Economic Freedom, 1994), p. 92.
10. Thomas Szasz, *The Theology of Medicine: The Political-Philosophical Foundations of Medical Ethics* [1977] (Syracuse: Syracuse University Press, 1988); *Pharmacracy: Medicine and Politics in America* [1999] (Syracuse: Syracuse University Press, 2001).
11. Henry Maudsley, *Responsibility in Mental Disease*, fourth edition (London: Kegan Paul, Trench & Co., 1885), pp. viii, 133, emphasis added.
12. Michael S. Moore, "Some myths about 'mental illness,'" *Archives of General Psychiatry*, 32: 1483-1497 (December), 1975; p. 1495.
13. Ludwig von Mises, *Human Action*, 1949 edition, op. cit., pp. 16, 18, emphasis added.
14. Ibid., p. 149, emphasis added.
15. Ludwig von Mises, *Omnipotent Government: The Rise of the Total State and Total War* [1944] (Spring Mills, PA: Libertarian Press, 1985), p. 52.
16. Ludwig von Mises, *Human Action*, 1949 edition, op. cit., p. 185.
17. Ibid., pp. 185-186.

18.   Ibid., p. 185, emphasis added.
19.   Ibid., p. 316, emphasis added.
20.   Ludwig von Mises, *Liberalism: A Socio-Economic Exposition* [1927], translated by Ralph Raico, edited by Arthur Goddard (Kansas City: Sheed Andrews and McMeel, 1978), p. 13, emphasis added.
21.   Ibid., pp. 14-15, emphasis added.
22.   Ibid., pp. 52-53.
23.   Ibid., pp. 54-55.
24.   Ludwig von Mises, *Human Action*, 1949 edition, op. cit., pp. 728-729, emphasis added.
25.   Thomas Szasz, *Our Right to Drugs: The Case for a Free Market* [1992] (Syracuse: Syracuse University Press, 1996).
26.   Ludwig von Mises, *Liberalism*, op. cit., p. 303.
27.   Ibid., pp. 192-193.
28.   This volume, chapter 11.
29.   Ludwig von Mises, *The Ultimate Foundations of Economic Science* (Princeton, NJ: D. Van Nostrand, 1962), p. 5.
30.   Ibid., p. 55, emphasis added.
31.   Ludwig von Mises, *Human Action*, 1949 edition, op. cit., p. 874.

Chapter 11. Friedrich von Hayek

1.   Albert Venn Dicey, *Lectures on the Relations between Law and Public Opinion in England During the Nineteenth Century* [1905, 1914], 2nd edition (London: Macmillan, 1963), p. lxxix.
2.   Ibid., p. li.
3.   Friedrich A. Hayek, *The Constitution of Liberty* (Chicago: University of Chicago Press, 1960), p. 206, emphasis added.
4.   Thomas Szasz, *Ceremonial Chemistry: The Ritual Persecution of Drugs, Addicts, and Pushers* [1976] (Syracuse: Syracuse University Press, 2003); *Our Right to Drugs: The Case for a Free Market* [1992] (Syracuse: Syracuse University Press, 1996).
5.   This volume, chapter 10.
6.   Friedrich A. Hayek, *The Constitution of Liberty*, op. cit., p. 18.
7.   Ibid., p. 77; emphasis added.
8.   Friedrich A. Hayek, *The Counter-Revolution of Science: Studies on the Abuse of Reason* (New York: The Free Press of Glencoe/Macmillan, 1955), p. 26.
9.   Alan Ebenstein, *Friedrich Hayek: A Biography* (New York: Palgrave, 2001), p. 13.
10.   Thomas Szasz, *Insanity: The Idea and Its Consequences* [1987] (Syracuse: Syracuse University Press, 1997).
11.   Thomas Szasz, *A Lexicon of Lunacy: Metaphoric Malady, Moral Responsibility, and Psychiatry* (New Brunswick, NJ: Transaction Publishers, 1993), and *Insanity*, op. cit.
12.   Friedrich A. Hayek, *The Constitution of Liberty*, op. cit., p. 78.
13.   Ibid., pp. 153-154, emphasis added.
14.   Thomas Szasz, *Anti-Freud: Karl Kraus's Criticism of Psychoanalysis and Psychiatry* [1976] (Syracuse: Syracuse University Press, 1990).
15.   Alan Ebenstein, *Friedrich Hayek*, op. cit., p. 37.
16.   Ibid., p. 213.
17.   Ibid., pp. 251-252.

18. Ibid., p. 303.

19. Josh Billings: "It is better to know nothing than to know what ain't so." In, *Bartlett's Familiar Quotations*, edited by Justin Kaplan, Sixteenth Edition (Boston: Little, Brown & Co., 1992), p. 479.

20. Friedrich A. Hayek, *The Sensory Order: An Inquiry Into the Foundations of Theoretical Psychology* [1952] (Chicago: University of Chicago Press, 1963).

21. Ibid., pp. 5, 53.

22. Ibid., p. 194.

23. Alan Ebenstein, *Friedrich Hayek*, op. cit., p. 148, emphasis added.

24. George H. Mead, *Mind, Self & Society: From the Standpoint of a Social Behaviorist*, edited by Charles W. Morris (Chicago: University of Chicago Press, 1934).

25. Cited in Alan Ebenstein, *Friedrich Hayek*, op. cit., p. 150, emphasis added.

26. Ibid.

27. Thomas Szasz, "Introduction," in *The Analysis of Sensations, and the Relation of the Physical to the Psychical*, by Ernst Mach, translated from the first German edition by C. M. Williams; revised and supplemented from the fifth German edition by S. Waterlow (New York: Dover, 1959), pp. v-xxxi.

28. Ernst Mach, *The Analysis of Sensations*, op. cit., p. xxvii.

29. Thomas Szasz, *Pain and Pleasure: A Study of Bodily Feelings* [1957], Second expanded edition [1975] (Syracuse: Syracuse University Press, 1988).

30. Thomas Szasz, *The Myth of Mental Illness: Foundations of a Theory of Personal Conduct* (New York: Hoeber-Harper, 1961); revised edition (New York: HarperCollins, 1974); *The Meaning of Mind: Language, Morality, and Neuroscience* [1996] (Syracuse: Syracuse University Press, 2002).

31. Friedrich A. Hayek, *The Counter-Revolution of Science*, op. cit., pp. 16, 26.

32. Oskar Morgenstern and John Von Neumann, *Theory of Games and Economic Behavior* (Princeton: Princeton University Press, 1944).

33. Friedrich A. Hayek, *Hayek on Hayek: An Autobiographical Dialogue*, edited by Stephen Kresge and Leif Wenar (Chicago: University of Chicago Press, 1994), p. 148.

34. Friedrich A. Hayek, "Friedrich August von Hayek's speech at the Nobel Banquet," December 10, 1974. *Les Prix Nobel, 1974*, emphasis added. http://www.nobel.se/economics/laureates/1974/hayek-speech.html

35. Friedrich A. Hayek, "The pretense of knowledge," Nobel Lectures, December 11, 1974, *Les Prix Nobel, 1974*, emphasis added. http://www.nobel.se/economics/laureates/1974/hayek-lecture.html

36. Thomas Szasz, *Pharmacracy: Medicine and Politics in America* [2001] (Syracuse: Syracuse University Press, 2003).

Chapter 12. Murray N. Rothbard

1. Llewellyn H. Rockwell, Jr., "Murray N. Rothbard: A Legacy of Liberty," February 20, 2003. http://www.mises.org/mnr.asp

2. Thomas Szasz, "Mises and psychiatry," *Liberty*, 16: 23-26 (February), 2002.

3. Thomas Szasz, *The Myth of Mental Illness: Foundations of a Theory of Personal Conduct* [1961], revised edition (New York: HarperCollins, 1974).

4. Murray Rothbard, "Rothbard on Szasz," http://www.lewrockwell.com, January 15, 2002.

5. Murray N. Rothbard, "Psychoanalysis as a weapon," Keynote Address at a conference—titled "Asclepius at Syracuse: Thomas Szasz, Libertarian Humanist"—sponsored by The Institute for Humanistic Studies, State University of New York at

Albany, M. E. Grenander, director, April 17-19, 1980. Rothbard's comments are excerpted from pp. 333-350 of the conference proceedings. http://www.lewrock-well.com, January 17 and 20, 2002; also at http://www.szasz.com.

6.   Murray N. Rothbard, *For a New Liberty: The Libertarian Manifesto* [1973], Revised Edition (New York: Collier, 1978), pp. 90, 92.
7.   Ibid., p. 318.
8.   Ibid., pp. 90, 93.
9.   http://www.szasz.com/ia/szasz/rothbard.html
10.   Chapter 10, on Branden.
11.   Justin Raimondo, *An Enemy of the State: The Life of Murray N. Rothbard* (Amherst, NY: Prometheus Books, 2000), pp. 295-296.
12.   Ibid.
13.   Ibid.

Chapter 13. Robert Nozick

1.   Christopher Lehmann-Haupt, "Robert Nozick, Harvard political philosopher, dies at 63," *New York Times*, January 24, 2002. http://www.nytimes.com/2002/01/24/obituaries/24NOZI.html.
2.   Robert Nozick, *Anarchy, State, and Utopia* (New York: Basic Books, 1974), p. ix-x.
3.   Ibid., p. ix.
4.   Ibid., pp. 338, 358, 348.
5.   Erving Goffman, *Asylums: Essays on the Social Situation of Mental Patients and Other Inmates* (Garden City, NY: Doubleday Anchor, 1961).
6.   Thomas Szasz, "American Association for the Abolition of Involuntary Mental Hospitalization," (Letter), *American Journal of Psychiatry*, 127: 1698 (June), 1971; and "The American Association for the Abolition of Involuntary Mental Hospitalization," *The Abolitionist,* 1: 1-2 (Summer), 1971. See also http://www.szasz.com.
7.   Helmut Schoeck and James W. Wigging, editors, *Psychiatry and Responsibility* (Princeton: D. Van Nostrand, 1962); Thomas Szasz, "Psychiatry as a Social Institution," in ibid., pp. 1-18.
8.   Robert Nozick, *Anarchy, State, and Utopia*, op. cit., p. 34.
9.   Ibid., p. 58, emphasis in the original.
10.   Ibid., p. 142.
11.   Ibid., p. 145.
12.   Ibid., pp. 35, 37.
13.   Peter Singer, *Practical Ethics*, 2nd edition (Cambridge: Cambridge University Press, 1993), and *Rethinking Life and Death: The Collapse of Our Traditional Ethics* (New York: St. Martin's Griffin, 1996). See also, Thomas Szasz, "The 'medical ethics' of Peter Singer," *Society*, 38: 20-25 (July/August), 2001.
14.   Robert Nozick, *Philosophical Explanations* (Cambridge: Harvard University Press, 1981), pp. 616-617.
15.   Ibid., p. 660.
16.   Ibid., p. 2, emphasis added.
17.   Robert Nozick, "Coercion," in Sidney Morgenbesser, Patrick Suppes, and Morton White, editors, *Philosophy, Science, and Method: Essays in Honor of Ernest Nagel* (New York: St. Martin's Press, 1969), pp. 440-472; p. 440.
18.   Ibid., p. 441.
19.   David Martin, "The ideal observers," *TLS*, February 7, 2003, pp. 3-4; p. 3.

20. Robert Nozick, "Coercion," op. cit., p. 579.
21. Viktor E. Frankl, *Viktor Frankl Recollections—An Autobiography* [1995], translated by Joseph Fabry and Judith Fabry (New York: Plenum Press, 1997). See also, Thomas Szasz, *The Myth of Psychotherapy: Mental Healing as Rhetoric, Religion, and Repression* [1978] (Syracuse University Press, 1988), p. 205; and Reuven P. Bulka, "Is logotherapy authoritarian?" *Journal of Humanistic Psychology*, 18: 45-54 (Fall), 1978; Rollo May, "Response to Bulka's article," ibid., p. 55; and Viktor Frankl, "Comment on Bulka's article," ibid., pp. 57-58.
22. Viktor Frankl, "'Nothing but'—On reductionism & nihilism," *Encounter* (London), 33: pp. 51-56, 1969; p. 55.
23. Benjamin Wilkomirski, *Fragments: Memories of a Wartime Childhood* [1995], translated by Carol Brown Janeway (New York: Schocken, 1996).
24. Cited in S. Friedlander, "True believers: Greed, ideology, power, and lust as motives for the Holocaust," *TLS* (*Times Literary Supplement*, London), March 1, 2002, pp. 4-6; pp. 5-6.
25. Robert Nozick, *The Examined Life: Philosophical Meditations* (New York: Simon and Schuster, 1989).
26. Ibid., pp. 16-17.
27. Ibid., pp. 25-26, emphasis added.
28. Ibid., p. 2.
29. Albert Camus, *The Myth of Sisyphus*, in *The Myth of Sisyphus, and Other Essays* [1942], translated by Justin O'Brien (New York: Vintage, 1955), p. 1.
30. *Compassion in Dying v. State of Wash.*, 79 F.3d 790 (9th Cir. 1996).
31. Thomas Szasz, *Fatal Freedom: The Ethics and Politics of Suicide* [1999] (Syracuse: Syracuse University Press, 2002).
32. *Quill v. Vacco*, 80 F.3d 716 (2nd Cir.) 1996, pp. 716-743; p. 721, emphasis added.
33. Thomas Szasz, *Fatal Freedom*, op. cit., pp. 1-2.
34. Deirdre McCloskey, *Crossing: A Memoir* (Chicago: University of Chicago Press, 1999); see this volume, chapter 15.
35. Ronald Dworkin, "Assisted suicide: The philosophers' brief," *New York Review of Books*, March 27, 1997, pp. 41-47; pp. 41, 43.
36. Ibid., p. 43, emphasis added.
37. Ibid., emphasis added.
38. Linda Genhouse, "Court, 9-0, upholds state laws prohibiting assisted suicide: No help for dying," *New York Times*, June 27, 1997, pp. A1 & A19.
39. Robert Nozick, *The Examined Life*, op. cit., p. 57.
40. Ibid., p. 67.
41. This volume, chapter 10.
42. Robert Nozik, *The Examined Life*, op. cit., p. 214, emphasis added.
43. Ibid., 287.
44. Ibid., p. 288, emphasis in the original.
45. Thomas Szasz, *Liberation By Oppression: A Comparative Study of Slavery and Psychiatry* (New Brunswick, NJ: Transaction Publishers, 2002); see also, *Cruel Compassion: The Psychiatric Control of Society's Unwanted* [1994] (Syracuse University Press, 1998).
46. Ibid., p. 284-285.
47. Robert Nozick, *The Nature of Rationality* (Princeton: Princeton University Press, 1993).
48. Ibid., pp. 26-27, emphasis in the original.
49. Ibid., p. 27, emphasis in the original.

50. Christopher Lehmann-Haupt, op. cit.; Robert Nozick, *Invariances: The Structure of the Objective World* (Cambridge: Harvard University Press, 2001).
51. Robert Nozick, *The Nature of Rationality*, op. cit, p. 295, emphasis added.
52. Colin McGinn, "An ardent fallibilist," *The New York Review of Books*, June 27, 2002, pp. 39-41; p. 39.
53. Quoted in ibid., p. 41, emphasis in the original.
54. Ibid., p. 41.
55. Ken Gewertz, "Philosopher Nozick dies at 63," *Harvard University Gazette*, January 23, 2002.
56. http://mbb.harvard.edu/MBB_ROOT/working_groups/default.html

Chapter 14. Julian Simon

1. Stephen Moore, "Julian Simon remembered: It's a wonderful life," *Cato Online Policy Report*, March/April, 1998. http://www.cato.org/pubs/policy_report/cpr-20n2-1.html; for Simon's views on foreign aid, see Julian Simon, "Population growth, economic growth, and foreign aid," *The Cato Journal*, 7: 159-186 (Spring/Summer), 1987.
2. Julian Simon, *Good Mood: The New Psychology of Overcoming Depression*, Foreword by Albert Ellis (LaSalle, IL: Open Court, 1993).
3. Ibid., p. 3.
4. Ibid.
5. Ibid.
6. Ibid., p. 13, emphasis added.
7. See Thomas Szasz, *The Myth of Psychotherapy: Mental Healing as Religion, Rhetoric, and Repression* [1978] (Syracuse: Syracuse University Press, 1988).
8. Julian Simon, *Good Mood*, op. cit., p. 43, emphasis in the original.
9. Ibid., p. 68, emphasis added.
10. Ibid., p. 102.
11. Ibid., p. 165.
12. Ibid., pp. 201-207.
13. Ibid., p. 246.
14. Ibid., p. 248.
15. Ibid., p. 250, emphasis added.
16. Ibid., p 251.
17. Albert Ellis Institute. "Albert Ellis Institute offering Rational Emotive Behavior Therapy (REBT)," www.rebt.org.
18. http://www.quotemeonit.com/reynolds.html
19. Rita J. Simon, "The Legitimacy of the Defense of Insanity," in Jeffrey Schaler, editor, *Szasz Under Fire* (Chicago: Open Court, in press), pp. xx; and Rita J. Simon and David E. Aaronson, *The Insanity Defense: A Critical Assessment of Law and Policy in the Post-Hinckley Era* (New York: Praeger, 1988).
20. See Thomas Szasz, "Reply to Rita Simon," in Jeffrey Schaler, editor, *Szasz Under Fire*, op. cit., in press.

Chapter 15. Deirdre N. McCloskey

1. Henry Herbert, Second Earl of Pembroke, in *Oxford Dictionary of Quotations*, 4th ed., edited by Angela Partington (New York: Oxford University Press, 1992), p. 511. The statement is also attributed to Jean-Louis de Lolme (1741-1806), a Geneva-born Calvinist lawyer and legal scholar and admirer of English Parliamentary

government: "It is a fundamental principle with English lawyers, that Parliament can do everything but make a woman a man, and a man a woman." Quoted in, Albert V. Dicey, *Introduction to the Study of the Law of the Constitution* [1885], 8th edition [1915], Foreword by Roger Michener (Indianapolis: Liberty Fund, 1982), p. 5.

2.   Gilbert K. Chesterton, *Heretics* [1905], p.143, in *G. K. Chesterton's Works on the Web*, http://www.dur.ac.uk/martin.ward/gkc/books/.

3.   Deirdre N. McCloskey, *Knowledge and Persuasion in Economics* (Cambridge: Cambridge University Press, 1994); *The Rhetoric of Economics (Rhetoric of the Human Sciences)*, 2nd edition (Madison, WI: University of Wisconsin Press, 1998); *Economical Writings*, 2nd edition (Prospect Heights, IL: Waveland Press, 1999); and *Crossing: A Memoir* (Chicago: University of Chicago Press, 1999). For a discussion of McCloskey's contributions to the critique of economic scientism and the rhetoric of economics, see chapter 10.

4.   Deirdre N. McCloskey, *Crossing*, op. cit., p. 7.

5.   Ibid., p. 43.

6.   Ibid.

7.   Ibid., p. 55, emphasis in the original.

8.   Ibid., p. 57, emphasis added.

9.   Ibid., p. 71.

10.   See Thomas Szasz, *Sex By Prescription: The Startling Truth about Today's Sex Therapy* [1980] (Syracuse: Syracuse University Press, 1990); also "Male women, female men," *New Republic*, October 9, 1976, pp. 8-9, reprinted in Thomas Szasz, *The Therapeutic State: Psychiatry in the Mirror of Current Events* (Buffalo: Prometheus Books, 1984), pp. 325-326; and "Male and female created He them," review of *The Transsexual Empire: The Making of the She-Male*, by Janice G. Raymond, the *New York Times Book Review*, June 10, 1979, pp. 11, 39, reprinted in Thomas Szasz, *The Therapeutic State*, op. cit., pp. 327-329.

11.   Deirdre N. McCloskey, *Crossing*, op. cit., 72.

12.   Ibid., pp. 72-73, 96-97, emphasis in the original.

13.   Ibid., emphasis in the original.

14.   See Thomas Szasz, *Liberation By Oppression: A Comparative Study of Slavery and Psychiatry* (New Brunswick, NJ: Transaction Publishers, 2002).

15.   Ibid., p. 98.

16.   Erving Goffman, *Asylums: Essays on the Social Situation of Mental Patients and Other Inmates* (Garden City, N.Y.: Doubleday Anchor, 1961), p.140.

17.   Deirdre N. McCloskey, *Crossing*, op. cit., p. 99, emphasis in the original.

18.   Ibid., pp. 106-109.

19.   Ibid., p. 113.

20.   Ibid., p. 115.

21.   Ibid., 117, emphasis in the original.

22.   Ibid., pp. 225, 226.

23.   Deirdre McCloskey, E-mail to Thomas Szasz, April 19, 2002.

24.   Ibid.

25.   Thomas Szasz, "Male and female created He them," op. cit.

26.   See Thomas Szasz, *Sex By Prescription*, op. cit., p. 74. Such an operation is alluded to in 1 Corinthians, 7:17-18.

27.   Thomas Szasz, *Insanity: The Idea and Its Consequences* [1987] (Syracuse: Syracuse University Press, 1997) and *Liberation By Oppression*, op. cit.

28.   Carl Elliott, *Better Than Well: American Medicine Meets the American Dream* (New York: Norton, 2003), p. 180.

29.   Maxine Kumin, "The metamorphosis," *New York Times*, November 14, 1999.

30. Deirdre McCloskey, "E-mail to Thomas Szasz," April 19, 2002 and iowa-mhcrc. psychiatry.uiowa.edu/new/MHCRC_Web_Page/genetics.html.

31. Ibid.

32. Maxine Kumin, "The metamorphosis," op. cit.

33. Jan Morris, *Conundrum: From James to Jan—An Extraordinary Personal Narrative* (New York: Harcourt Brace Jovanovich, 1974).

34. See for example, Roberta Cowell, *Roberta Cowell's Story: An Autobiography* (London: Heinemann, 1954); Christine Jorgensen, *Christine Jorgensen: A Personal Autobiography* (New York: Paul Eriksson, 1967); Michael Vitez, "Their love survived great changes," *Philadelphia Inquirer*, January 9, 2003. http://www.hrc. org/familynet /newsstand.asp?ID=1911

35. Ann Hodges, "Love conquers all in HBO's risky film 'Normal'," *Houston Chronicle*, March 17, 2003. http://www.chron.com/cs/CDA/story.hts/ae/tv/1817321

36. A. J. Frutkin, "Film asks, What aspect of a person do you love?" *Washington Post*, March 16, 2003, p. Y7. http://www.washingtonpost.com/wp-dyn/articles/ A12803-2003Mar11.html

37. Marjorie King, "Queering the schools," *City Journal*, Spring 2003, Vol. 13, No. 2. http://www.city-journal.org/html/13_2_queering_the_schools.html

38. Anton Pavlovich Chekhov, *Ward No. 6*, in Thomas Szasz, editor, *The Age of Madness: A History of Involuntary Mental Hospitalization Presented in Selected Texts* (Garden City, NY: Doubleday Anchor, 1973), p. 101.

39. There is a vast literature on this subject. See for example John Macmurray, *Persons in Relation* (London: Faber and Faber, 1961); C. B. Macpherson, *The Political Theory of Possessive Individualism: Hobbes to Locke* (London: Oxford University Press, 1962); George Herbert Mead, *Mind, Self, and Society: From the Standpoint of a Social Behaviorist*, edited by Charles W. Morris (Chicago: University of Chicago Press, 1934); Steven Lukes, *Individualism* (Oxford: Basil Blackwell, 1973); A. John Simmons, *Justification and Legitimacy: Essays on Rights and Obligations* (Cambridge: Cambridge University Press, 2001).

40. Henry Sumner Maine, *Ancient Law: Its Connection with the Early History of Society, and Its Relation to Modern Ideas* [1864], Foreword by Lawrence Rosen (Tucson: University of Arizona Press, 1986), p. 165, emphasis in the original.

41. Michael O. Hardimon, "Role obligations," *Journal of Philosophy* 91: 333-363, 1994.

42. Thomas Szasz, *Sex By Prescription*, op. cit.

43. American Psychiatric Association, *Diagnostic and Statistical Manual of Mental Disorders—IV-TR*, fourth edition, text revision (Washington, D.C.: American Psychiatric Association, 2000), pp. 576-580; p. 579.

44. http://www.blackwell-synergy.com/servletuseragent?func=synergy&synergy Action=showFullText&doi=10.1046 j.1440-1614.2001.00859.x

45. Benjamin James Sadock and Virginia Alcott Sadock, *Kaplan & Sadock's Synopsis of Psychiatry: Behavioral Sciences/Clinical Psychiatry*, ninth edition (Philadelphia: Lippincott Williams & Wilkins), 2003, p. 738.

46. For two dramatic examples, see Bernard Wasserstein, *The Secret Lives of Trebitsch Lincoln* (London: Penguin, 1989), and Francis Wheen, *Who Was Dr. Charlotte Bach?* (London: Short Books, 2002).

Finale

1. http://www.quotedb.com/quote.php?quoteid=1275. This line is often quoted but may be a false attribution.

Bibliography

Acton, John E.E.D. *Essays in the Study and Writing of History*, edited by J. Rufus Fears, 3 vols. (Indianapolis: Liberty Classics, 1988).

Adler, Mortimer J. *The Idea of Freedom*, 2 vols. (Garden City, NY: Doubleday, 1958-1961).

Aeschliman, Michael D. *The Restitution of Man: C. S. Lewis and the Case Against Scientism* (Grand Rapids, MI: William B. Eerdmans Publishing Company, 1983).

American Psychiatric Association, *Diagnostic and Statistical Manual of Mental Disorders—IV*, Fourth Edition (Washington, D.C.: American Psychiatric Association, 1994).

American Psychiatric Association, *Diagnostic and Statistical Manual of Mental Disorders—IV—TR*, Fourth Edition, Text Revision (Washington, D.C.: American Psychiatric Association, 2000).

Arendt, Hannah. *Between Past and Future: Six Exercises in Political Thought* [1954] (New York: Meridian, 1961).

Bailyn, Bernard. *To Begin the World Anew: The Genius and Ambiguities of the American Founders* (New York: Knopf, 2003).

Bauer, Peter T. *Dissent on Development: Studies and Debates in Development*, revised edition (Cambrdige: Harvard University Press, 1976).

Bauer, Peter T. *Equality, the Third World, and Economic Delusion* (London: Weidenfeld and Nicolson, 1981).

Bauer, Peter T. *Reality and Rhetoric: Studies in Economic Development* (London: Weidenfeld and Nicolson, 1984).

Bauer, Peter T. *From Subsistence to Exchange, and Other Essays* (Princeton: Princeton University Press, 2000).

Beck, James C., ed. *Confidentiality Versus the Duty to Protect: Foreseeable Harm in the Practice of Psychiatry* (Washington, D.C.: American Psychiatric Press, 1990).

Bergland, David. *Libertarianism in One Lesson* (Costa Mesa, CA: Orpheus Publications, 1984).

Black, H. C. *Black's Law Dictionary*, revised 4th edition (St. Paul: West, 1968).

Boaz, David. *Libertarianism: A Primer* (New York: Free Press, 1997).

Boaz, David, ed. *The Libertarian Reader: Classic and Contemporary Readings from Lao-Tzu to Milton Friedman* (New York: Free Press, 1997).

Boaz, David, ed. *Toward Liberty: The Idea that is Changing the World, 25 Years of Public Policy from the Cato Institute* (Washington, D.C.: Cato Institute, 2002).

Branden, Barbara. *The Passion of Ayn Rand* (New York: Doubleday, 1986).

Branden, Nathaniel. *The Psychology of Self-Esteem: A New Concept of Man's Psychological Nature* (Los Angeles: Nash, 1969).

Branden, Nathaniel. *Breaking Free* (Los Angeles: Nash, 1970).

Branden, Nathaniel. *Judgment Day: My Years with Ayn Rand* (Boston: Houghton Mifflin, 1989).

Buchanan, James M. *What Should Economists Do?* (Indianapolis: Liberty Press, 1979).

Burke, Edmund. *Reflections on the Revolution in France* [1790], Foreword by Francis Canavan (Indianapolis: Liberty Fund, 1999).

Burke, Edmund. *The Works of the Right Honorable Edmund Burke*, 12 vols. (Boston: Wells & Lilly, 1826).

Butler, Eamon. *Hayek: His Contributions to the Political and Economic Thought of Our Time* (London: Temple Smith, 1983).

Camus, Albert. *The Myth of Sisyphus*, in *The Myth of Sisyphus, and Other Essays* [1942], translated by Justin O'Brien (New York: Vintage, 1955).

Camus, Albert. *The Rebel: An Essay on Man in Revolt* [1951], translated by Anthony Bower (New York: Vintage Books, 1956).

Camus, Albert. *Resistance, Rebellion, and Death*, translated by Justin O'Brien (New York: Knopf, 1961).

Carpenter, Ted Galen. *Bad Neighbor Policy: Washington's Futile War on Drugs in Latin America* (New York: Palgrave, 2003).

Chekhov, Anton Pavlovich. *Ward No. 6*, in Thomas Szasz, editor, *The Age of Madness: A History of Involuntary Mental Hospitalization Presented in Selected Texts* (Garden City, NY: Doubleday Anchor, 1973), p. 101.

Chesterton, Gilbert K. *Orthodoxy* (London: John Lane, 1909).

Chesterton, Gilbert K. *What's Wrong with the World* (New York: Dodd, Mead and Company, 1910). http://www.ccel.org/c/chesterton/wrongworld/wrongworld.txt

Clay, John. *R. D. Laing: A Divided Self* (London: Hodder & Stoughton, 1996).

Crammer, John. *Asylum History: Buckinghamshire County Pauper Lunatic Asylum—St. John's* (London: Gaskell, 1990).

Danford, John W. *Roots of Freedom: A Primer on Modern Liberty* (Wilington, DE: ISI Books, 2000).

Dante Alighieri, *The Inferno*, translated by John Ciardi (New York: Mentor, 1954).

Dante Alighieri, *The Divine Comedy of Dante Alighieri*, translated by John D. Sinclair (New York: Oxford University Press, 1968).

Dicey, Albert V. *Introduction to the Study of the Law of the Constitution* [1885], 8th edition [1915], Foreword by Roger Michener (Indianapolis: Liberty Fund, 1982).

Dicey, Albert V. *Lectures on the Relation Between Law and Public Opinion in England During the Nineteenth Century*, 2nd edition (London: Macmillan, 1914).

Dolan, Edwin, ed. *The Foundations of Modern Austrian Economics* (Kansas City: Sheed and Ward, 1976).

Dorn, James A., Steven H. Hanke, and Alan A. Walters, eds. *The Revolution in Development Economics* (Washington, D.C.: Cato Institute, 1998).

Ebeling, Richard M. *Austrian Economics and the Political Economy of Freedom* (Northhampton, MA: Edward Elgar, 2003).

Ebenstein, Alan, William Ebenstein, and Edwin Fogelman, *Today's Isms: Socialism, Capitalism, Fascism, Communism, Libertarianism*, eleventh edition (Upper Saddle River, NJ: Prentice-Hall, 2000).

Edwards, Rem B., and Glenn C. Garber, eds. *Bio-Ethics* (New York: Harcourt Brace Jovanovich, 1988).

Egan, Kieran. *Getting It Wrong from the Beginning: Our Progressivist Inheritance from Herbert Spencer, John Dewey, and Jean Piaget* (New Haven: Yale University Press, 2002).

Einstein, Albert. *The World as I See It* (New York: Covici, Friede, 1934).

Ferguson, Niall. *The Cash Nexus: Money and Power in the Modern World, 1700-2000* (New York: Basic Books, 2001).

Ferris, Timothy, ed. *The World Treasury of Physics, Astronomy, and Mathematics* (Boston: Little, Brown and Company, 1991).

Fogel, Robert William. *Without Consent or Contract: The Rise and Fall of American Slavery* (New York: Norton, 1989).

Frankl, Viktor E. *Recollections—An Autobiography* [1995], translated by Joseph Fabry and Judith Fabry (New York: Plenum Press, 1997).

Freeman, Hugh, ed. *A Century of Psychiatry* (London: Mosby-Wolfe/Harcourt Publishers, 1999).

Freud, Sigmund. *The Standard Edition of the Complete Psychological Works of Sigmund Freud*, translated by James Strachey, 24 vols. (London: Hogarth Press, 1953-1974).

Friedman, David. *The Machinery of Freedom: Guide to Radical Capitalism*, second edition (LaSalle, IL: Open Court, 1989).

Friedman, Milton. *Capitalism and Freedom* (Chicago: University of Chicago Press, 1962).

Goffman, E. *Asylums: Essays on the Social Situation of Mental Patients and Other Inmates* (Garden City, NY: Doubleday Anchor, 1961).

Gottfried, Paul E. *After Liberalism: Mass Democracy in the Managerial State* (Princeton: Princeton University Press, 2001).

Gottfried, Paul E. *Multiculturalism and the Politics of Guilt* (Columbia, MO: University of Missouri Press, 2002).

Great Quotations, The, compiled by George Seldes (New York: Lyle Stuart, 1960).

Hayek, Friedrich A. *The Counter-Revolution of Science: Studies on the Abuse of Reason* (New York: The Free Press of Glencoe/Macmillan, 1955).

Hayek, Friedrich A. *The Constitution of Liberty* (Chicago: University of Chicago Press, 1960).

Hayek, Friedrich A. *The Fatal Conceit: The Errors of Socialism*, edited by W. W. Bartley, III (Chicago: University of Chicago Press, 1989).

Hayek, Friedrich A. *Hayek on Hayek: An Autobiographical Dialogue*, edited by Stephen Kresge and Leif Wenar (Chicago: University of Chicago Press, 1994).

Herrnstein, Richard J. and Charles Murray, *The Bell Curve: Intelligence and Class Structure in American Life* (New York: Free Press, 1994).

Higgs, Robert. *Crisis and Leviathan: Critical Episodes in the Growth of American Government* (New York: Oxford University Press, 1987).

Hoppe, Hans-Hermann. *A Theory of Socialism and Capitalism: Economics, Politics, and Ethics* (Boston: Kluwer Academic Publishers, 1989).

Hoppe, Hans-Hermann. *Democracy—The God That Failed: The Economics and Politics of Monarchy, Democracy, and Natural Order* (New Brunswick, NJ: Transaction Publishers, 2001).

Hospers, John. *Libertarianism: A Political Philosophy for Tomorrow* (Los Angeles: Nash Publishing, 1971).

Hume, David. *Hume's Ethical Writings: Selections from David Hume*, edited and with an Introduction by Alasdair MacIntyre (Notre Dame, IN: University of Notre Dame Press, 1965).

Jay, Anthony, ed. *The Oxford Dictionary of Political Quotations* (New York: Oxford University Press, 1996).

Jones, Ernest. *The Life and Work of Sigmund Freud*, 3 vols. (New York: Basic Books, 1953-1957).

Kaplan, Justin, ed. *Bartlett's Familiar Quotations*, Sixteenth Edition (Boston: Little, Brown & Co., 1992).

Keane, John. *Tom Paine: A Political Life* (London: Bloomsbury, 1995).

Keynes, John Maynard. *The General Theory of Employment, Interest, and Money* (New York: Harcourt, Brace, 1936).

Kimball, Roger. *Experiments Against Reality: The Fate of Culture in the Postmodern Age* (Chicago: Ivan Dee, 2000).

Klein, Donald F. and Paul H. Wender, *Understanding Depression: A Complete Guide to Its Diagnosis and Treatment* (New York: Oxford University Press, 1993).

Laing, Ronald D. *The Divided Self: An Existential Study in Sanity and Madness* (London: Tavistock Publications, 1960).

Laing, Ronald D. *The Politics of Experience and the Bird of Paradise* (Harmondsworth: Penguin, 1967).

Letwin, Shirley Robin. *The Pursuit of Certainty: David Hume, Jeremy Bentham, John Stuart Mill, Beatrice Webb* [1965] (Indianapolis: Liberty Fund, 1998).

Levy, Robert M. and Leonard S. Rubenstein, *The Rights of People with Mental Disabilities: The Authoritative ACLU Guide to the Rights of People with Mental Illness and Mental Retardation* (Carbondale, IL: Southern Illinois University Press, 1996).

Locke, John. *An Essay Concerning Human Understanding* [1690] (Chicago: Regnery/Gateway, 1956).

Locke, John. *Two Treatises on Government* [1690], edited by Peter Laslett (New York: New American Library, 1965).

Lukes, Steven. *Individualism* (Oxford: Basil Blackwell, 1973).

Macfarlane, Alan. *The Origins of English Individualism: The Family, Property and Social Transition* (Oxford: Basil Blackwell, 1978).

Machan, Tibor R. *The Libertarian Alternative: Essays in Social and Political Philosophy* (Chicago: Nelson-Hall, 1974).

Machan, Tibor R., ed. *The Libertarian Reader* (Totowa, NJ: Rowman and Littlefield, 1982).

Machan, Tibor R. and Douglas B. Rasmussen, eds. *Liberty for the Twenty-first Century: Contemporary Libertarian Thought* (Lanham, MD: Rowman & Littlefield, 1995).

Machlup, Fritz, ed. *Essays on Hayek* (New York: New York University Press, 1976).

Macmurray, John. *Persons in Relation* (London: Faber and Faber, 1961).

Macmurray, John. *The Self as Agent* [1957] (London: Faber and Faber, 1969).

Macpherson, C. B. *The Political Theory of Possessive Individualism: Hobbes to Locke* (London: Oxford University Press, 1962).

Maine, Henry Sumner. *Ancient Law: Its Connection with the Early History of Society, and Its Relation to Modern Ideas* [1864], foreword by Lawrence Rosen (Tucson: University of Arizona Press, 1986).

Manning, Philip. *Erving Goffman and Modern Sociology* (Stanford, CA: Stanford University Press, 1992).

McCloskey, Deirdre N. *Crossing: A Memoir* (Chicago: University of Chicago Press, 1999).

McCloskey, Donald (Deirdre) N. *The Rhetoric of Economics* (Madison: University of Wisconsin Press, 1985).

McLeod, Hugh. *Secularisation in Western Europe, 1848-1914* (New York: St. Martin's Press, 2000).

Mead, George Herbert. *Mind, Self, and Society: From the Standpoint of a Social Behaviorist*, edited by Charles W. Morris (Chicago: University of Chicago Press, 1934).

Menninger, Karl. *The Vital Balance: The Life Process in Mental Health and Illness* (New York: Viking, 1963).

Menninger, Karl. *The Crime of Punishment* (New York: Viking, 1968).

Merton, Robert K. *Social Theory and Social Structure* [1949], enlarged edition (New York: Free Press, 1968).

Meyerowitz, Joanne. *How Sex Changed: A History of Transsexuality in the United States* (Cambridge: Harvard University Press, 2003).

Meynert, Theodor. *Psychiatry: Clinical Treatise on Diseases of the Forebrain* [1884], translated by B. Sachs (New York: G. P. Putnam's Sons, 1885).

Mill, John Stuart. *On Liberty* [1859] (Chicago: Regnery, 1955).

Mill, John Stuart. *Utilitarianism* [1863], in *Essential Works of John Stuart Mill*, edited by Max Lerner (New York: Bantam Books, 1961).

Mill, John Stuart. *Literary Essays*, edited by Edward Alexander (Indianapolis: Bobbs-Merrill, 1967).

Mill, John Stuart. *Collected Works of John Stuart Mill*, edited by Ann P. Robson and John M. Brown, 25 vols. (Toronto: University of Toronto Press, 1986).

Minogue, Kenneth R. *The Liberal Mind* (London: Methuen, 1963).

Minogue, Kenneth R. *Alien Powers: The Pure Theory of Ideology* (New York: St. Martin's Press, 1985).

Mises, Ludwig von. *Human Action: A Treatise on Economics* (New Haven: Yale University Press, 1949).

Mises, Ludwig von. *The Ultimate Foundations of Economic Science* (Princeton, NJ: D. Van Nostrand, 1962).

Mises, Ludwig von. *Liberalism: A Socio-Economic Exposition* [1927], translated by Ralph Raico, edited by Arthur Goddard (Kansas City: Sheed Andrews and McMeel, 1978).

Mises, Ludwig von. *Socialism: An Economic and Sociological Analysis* [1922], translated from the second German edition [1932] by J. Kahane (Indianapolis: Liberty Classics, 1981).

Mises, Ludwig von. *Omnipotent Government: The Rise of the Total State and Total War* [1944] (Spring Mills, PA: Libertarian Press, 1985).

Morgenstern, Oskar and John von Neumann. *Theory of Games and Economic Behavior* (Princeton: Princeton University Press, 1944).

Morse, Jennifer Roback. *Love & Economics: Why the Laissez-Faire Family Doesn't Work* (Dallas: Pence Publishing Company, 2001).

Murray, Charles. *Losing Ground: American Social Policy, 1950-1980* (New York: Basic Books, 1984).

Murray, Charles. *What It Means to Be a Libertarian: A Personal Interpretation* (New York: Broadway Books, 1997).

Narveson, Jan. *The Libertarian Idea* (Philadelphia: Temple University Press, 1988).

Neier, Aryeh. *Taking Liberties: Four Decades in the Struggle for Rights* (New York: Public Affairs, 2003).

Nelson, Robert H. *Reaching for Heaven on Earth: The Theological Meaning of Economics* (Lanham, MD: Rowman and Littlefield, 1991).

Nelson, Robert H. *Economics as Religion: From Samuelson to Chicago and Beyond* (University Park: Pennsylvania State University Press, 2001).

Nishiyama, Chiaki and Kurt R. Leube, eds. *The Essence of Hayek* (Stanford, CA: Hoover Institution Press, 1984).

Nock, Albert Jay. *Our Enemy, The State* (New York: William Morrow, 1935).

Nock, Albert Jay. *Memoirs of a Superfluous Man* [1943] (Chicago: Regnery, 1964).

Nock, Albert Jay. *The State of the Union: Essays in Social Criticism*, edited by Charles H. Hamilton (Indianapolis: Liberty Fund, 1991).

Nozick, Robert. *Anarchy, State, and Utopia* (New York: Basic Books, 1974).

Nozick, Robert. *Philosophical Explanations* (Cambridge: Harvard University Press, 1981).

Nozick, Robert. *The Examined Life: Philosophical Meditations* (New York: Simon and Schuster, 1989).

Nozick, Robert. *The Nature of Rationality* (Princeton: Princeton University Press, 1993).

Opitz, Edmund A. *The Libertarian Theology of Freedom* (Tampa, FL: Hallberg Publishing Corporation, 1999).

Peirce, Charles S., *Values in a Universe of Chance: Selected Writings of Charles S. Peirce (1839-1914)*, edited by Philip P. Wiener (Garden City, NY: Doubleday Anchor, 1958).

Polanyi, Michael. *Personal Knowledge: Towards a Post-Critical Philosophy* (Chicago: University of Chicago Press, 1958).

Polanyi, Michael. *Knowing and Being: Essays by Michael Polanyi*, edited by Marjorie Greene (Chicago: University of Chicago Press, 1968).

Powell, Jim. *The Triumph of Liberty: A 2,000-Year History, Told Through the Lives of Freedom's Greatest Champions* (New York: Free Press, 2000).

Raeder, Linda. *John Stuart Mill and the Religion of Humanity* (Columbia, MO: University of Missouri Press, 2002).

Raimondo, Justin. *An Enemy of the State: The Life of Murray N. Rothbard* (Amherst, NY: Prometheus Books, 2000).

Rand, Ayn. *Letters of Ayn Rand,* edited by Michael S. Berliner, Introduction by Leonard Peikoff (New York: E. P. Dutton, 1995).

Reisman, George. *Capitalism: A Treatise on Economics* (Ottawa, Ill: Jameson Books, 1990).

Röpke, Wilhelm. *Welfare, Freedom and Inflation* (Tuscaloosa, AL: University of Alabama Press, 1964).

Röpke, Wilhelm. *A Humane Economy: The Special Framework of the Free Market* [1958] (Indianapolis: Liberty Fund, 1971).

Rothbard, Murray. *America's Great Depression* [1963] (Los Angeles: Nash, 1972).

Rothbard, Murray. *For a New Liberty: The Libertarian Manifesto* [1973], Revised Edition (New York: Collier, 1978).

Russell, Bertrand. *Roads to Freedom: Socialism, Anarchism, and Syndicalism* [1918] (London: George Allen and Unwin, 1966).

Russell, Bertrand. *The Conquest of Happiness* (New York: Horace Liveright, 1930).

Russell, Bertrand. *Power: A New Social Analysis* (London: George Allen & Unwin, 1938).

Russell, Bertrand. *Unpopular Essays* (New York: Simon & Schuster, 1950).

Russell, Bertrand. *Satan in the Suburbs, and Other Stories* (New York: Simon and Schuster, 1953).

Russell, Bertrand. *Nightmares of Eminent Persons, and Other Stories* [1954] (Harmondsworth: Penguin, 1962).

Sadock, Benjamin and Virginia Alcott Sadock. *Kaplan & Sadock's Synopsis of Psychiatry: Behavioral Sciences/Clinical Psychiatry,* ninth edition (Philadelphia: Lippincott Williams & Wilkins), 2003.

Samuelson, Paul A. *Foundations of Economic Analysis* (Harvard University Press, 1947).

Samuelson, Paul A. *Economics* (New York: McGraw-Hill, 1948).

Schaler, Jeffrey A., ed. *Szasz Under Fire* (Chicago: Open Court, 2004).

Schneewind, Jerome B., ed. *Mill's Ethical Writings* (New York: Collier/Macmillan, 1965).

Schneewind, Jerome B., ed. *Mill: A Collection of Critical Essays* (Garden City, NY: Anchor Books, 1968).

Schoeck, Helmut. *Envy: A Theory of Social Behaviour* [1966], translated by Michael Glenny and Betty Ross (New York: Harcourt, Brace & World, 1969).

Schoeck, Helmut and James W. Wigging, eds. *Psychiatry and Responsibility* (Princeton: D. Van Nostrand, 1962).

Sciabarra, Chris Matthew. *Ayn Rand: The Russian Radical* (University Park, PA: Pennsylvania State University Press, 1995).

Sciabarra, Chris Matthew. *Total Freedom: Toward a Dialectical Libertarianism* (University Park, PA: Pennsylvania State University Press, 2000).

Sen, Amartya. *Rationality and Freedom* (Cambridge: Harvard University Press, 2002).

Shutts, David. *Lobotomy: Resort to the Knife* (New York: Van Nostrand Reinhold, 1982).

Simmons, A. John. *Justification and Legitimacy: Essays on Rights and Obligations* (Cambridge: Cambridge University Press, 2001).

Simon, Julian. *Good Mood: The New Psychology of Overcoming Depression*, Foreword by Albert Ellis (LaSalle, IL: Open Court, 1993).

Simon, Rita J. and David E. Aaronson, *The Insanity Defense: A Critical Assessment of Law and Policy in the Post-Hinckley Era* (New York: Praeger, 1988).

Singer, Peter. *Practical Ethics*, 2nd edition (Cambridge: Cambridge University Press, 1993).

Singer, Peter. *Rethinking Life and Death: The Collapse of Our Traditional Ethics* (New York: St. Martin's Griffin, 1996).

Smith, Adam. *An Inquiry into the Nature and Causes of the Wealth of Nations* [1776], edited by Bruce Mazlish (Indianapolis: Bobbs-Merrill, 1961).

Smith, Adam. *The Theory of Moral Sentiments* [1759] (Indianapolis, IN: Liberty Classics, 1976).

Smith, Adam. *The Wisdom of Adam Smith*, selected by John Haggarty, edited by Benjamin A. Rogge John (Indianapolis, IN: Liberty Classics, 1976).

Smith, Adam. *The Wealth of Nations, Books I-III* [1776], Introduction by Andrew Skinner (London: Penguin, 1987).

Smith, Adam. *The Correspondence of Adam Smith*, edited by Ernest Campbell Mossner and Ian Simpson Ross (Indianapolis, IN: Liberty Classics, 1987).

Streissler, Erich, ed. *Roads to Freedom: Essays in Honour of Friedrich A. Von Hayek* (London: Routledge & Kegan Paul, 1976).

Sumner, William Graham. *What Social Classes Owe to Each Other* [1883] (Caldwell, ID: Caxton Publishers, 1963).

Sumner, William Graham. *On Liberty, Society, and Politics, The Essential Essays of William Graham Sumner*, edited by Robert C. Bannister (Indianapolis: Liberty Fund, 1992).

Sutherland, Stuart. *Irrationality: Why We Don't Think Straight!* (New Brunswick, NJ: Rutgers University Press, 1994).

Szasz, Thomas. *The Second Sin* (Garden City, NY: Doubleday Anchor, 1973).

Szasz, Thomas. *The Myth of Mental Illness: Foundations of a Theory of Personal Conduct* [1961], revised edition (New York: HarperCollins, 1974).

Szasz, Thomas. *The Therapeutic State: Psychiatry in the Mirror of Current Events.* (Buffalo: Prometheus Books, 1984).

Szasz, Thomas. *The Ethics of Psychoanalysis: The Theory and Method of Autonomous Psychotherapy* [1965] (Syracuse: Syracuse University Press, 1988).

Szasz, Thomas. *The Myth of Psychotherapy: Mental Healing as Religion, Rhetoric, and Repression* [1978] (Syracuse: Syracuse University Press, 1988).

Szasz, Thomas. *Pain and Pleasure: A Study of Bodily Feelings* [1957], second expanded edition [1975] (Syracuse: Syracuse University Press, 1988).

Szasz, Thomas. *Psychiatric Justice* [1965] (Syracuse: Syracuse University Press, 1988).

Szasz, Thomas. *Schizophrenia: The Sacred Symbol of Psychiatry* [1976] (Syracuse: Syracuse University Press, 1988).

Szasz, Thomas. *The Theology of Medicine: The Political-Philosophical Foundations of Medical Ethics* [1977] (Syracuse: Syracuse University Press, 1988).

Szasz, Thomas. *Law, Liberty, and Psychiatry: An Inquiry into the Social Uses of Psychiatry* [1963] (Syracuse: Syracuse University Press, 1989).

Szasz, Thomas. *Anti-Freud: Karl Kraus's Criticism of Psychoanalysis and Psychiatry* [1976] (Syracuse: Syracuse University Press, 1990).

Szasz, Thomas. *Sex By Prescription* [1980] (Syracuse: Syracuse University Press, 1990).

Szasz, Thomas. *Ideology and Insanity: Essays on the Psychiatric Dehumanization of Man* [1970] (Syracuse: Syracuse University Press, 1991).

Szasz, Thomas. *A Lexicon of Lunacy: Metaphoric Malady, Moral Responsibility, and Psychiatry* (New Brunswick, NJ: Transaction Publishers, 1993).

Szasz, Thomas. *Our Right to Drugs: The Case for a Free Market* [1992] (Syracuse: Syracuse University Press, 1996).

Szasz, Thomas. *Insanity: The Idea and Its Consequences* [1987] (Syracuse: Syracuse University Press, 1997).

Szasz, Thomas. *The Manufacture of Madness: A Comparative Study of the Inquisition and the Mental Health Movement* [1970] (Syracuse: Syracuse University Press, 1997).

Szasz, Thomas. *Cruel Compassion: The Psychiatric Control of Society's Unwanted* [1994] (Syracuse: Syracuse University Press, 1998).

Szasz, Thomas. *Psychiatric Slavery: When Confinement and Coercion Masquerade as Cure* [1977] (Syracuse: Syracuse University Press, 1998).

Szasz, Thomas. *Fatal Freedom: The Ethics and Politics of Suicide* [1999] (Syracuse: Syracuse University Press, 2002).

Szasz, Thomas. *Liberation By Oppression: A Comparative Study of Slavery and Psychiatry* (New Brunswick, NJ: Transaction Publishers, 2002).

Szasz, Thomas. *The Meaning of Mind: Language, Morality, and Neuroscience* [1996] (Syracuse: Syracuse University Press, 2002).

Szasz, Thomas. *Ceremonial Chemistry: The Ritual Persecution of Drugs, Addicts, and Pushers* [1976] (Syracuse: Syracuse University Press, 2003).

Szasz, Thomas. *Pharmacracy: Medicine and Politics in America* [2001] (Syracuse: Syracuse University Press, 2003).

Szasz, Thomas. *Words to the Wise: A Medical-Philosophical Dictionary* (Brunswick, NJ: Transaction Publishers, 2003).

Szasz, Thomas, ed. *The Age of Madness: A History of Involuntary Mental Hospitalization Presented in Selected Texts* (Garden City, NY: Doubleday Anchor, 1973).

Talmon, Jacob L. *The Origin of Totalitarian Democracy* (New York: Frederick A. Praeger, 1960).

Thornton, Bruce. *Plagues of the Mind: The New Epidemic of False Knowledge* (Wilmington, DE: ISI Books, 1999).

Tocqueville, A. de. *Democracy in America* [1835-40], edited by Phillips Bradley, 2 vols. (New York: Vintage, 1945).

Tocqueville, A. de. *Democracy in America* [1835-40], translated by Henry Reeve, edited by Henry Steele Commager (London: Oxford University Press, 1953).

Traupman, J. C. *The New College Latin & English Dictionary*. New York: Bantam, 1966.

Twight, Charlotte. *Dependent on D.C.: The Rise of Federal Control Over the Lives of Ordinary Americans* (New York: St. Martin's Press/Palgrave, 2002).

Veatch, Henry B. *Rational Man: A Modern Interpretation of Aristotelian Ethics* (Bloomington: Indiana University Press, 1962).

Walker, Jeff. *The Ayn Rand Cult* (Chicago: Open Court, 1999).

Wasserstein, Bernard. *The Secret Lives of Trebitsch Lincoln* (London : Penguin, 1989).

Weaver, Richard M. *Ideas Have Consequences* (Chicago: University of Chicago Press/Phoenix Books, 1962).

Weaver, Richard M. *Visions of Order: The Cultural Crisis of Our Time* (Baton Rouge, LA: Louisiana State University Press, 1964).

Webster, Charles. *From Paracelsus to Newton: Magic and the Making of Modern Science* [1982] (New York: Barnes & Noble, 1996).

Webster's Third New International Dictionary (Springfield, MA: G. & C. Merriam Co., 1961).

Weindling, Paul. *Health, Race and German Politics between National Unification and Nazism, 1870-1945* (Cambridge: Cambridge University Press, 1989).

Wertheimer, Alan. *Coercion* (Princeton: Princeton University Press, 1987).

West, Edwin G. *Adam Smith: The Man and His Works* (Indianapolis: Liberty Press, 1976).

West, Edwin G. *Education and the State: A Study in Political Economy*, third edition revised and expanded (Indianapolis: Liberty Press, 1994).

Wiener, Norbert. *God and Golem, Inc.: A Comment on Certain Points where Cybernetics Impinges on Religion* (Cambrdige: M.I.T. Press, 1964).

Wiener, Philip P., ed. *Dictionary of the History of Ideas*, 4 vols. (New York: Scribner's, 1973).

Wieser, Friedrich von. *Social Economics* [1914], translated by A. Ford Hinrichs (New York: Greenberg, 1927).

Wilkomirski, Benjamin. *Fragments: Memories of a Wartime Childhood* [1995], translated by Carol Brown Janeway (New York: Schocken, 1996).

Yeo, Richard. *Defining Science: William Whewell, Natural Knowledge, and Public Debate in Early Victorian England* (Cambridge: Cambridge University Press, 1993).

Index